PORTFOLIOS

for Nursing, Midwifery and other Health Professions 4e

PORTFOLIOS

for Nursing, Midwifery and other Health Professions 4e

Lynette Cusack and Morgan Smith

ELSEVIER

ELSEVIER

Elsevier Australia. ACN 001 002 357
(a division of Reed International Books Australia Pty Ltd)
Tower 1, 475 Victoria Avenue, Chatswood, NSW 2067

ISBN: 978-0-7295-4352-1

Notice

Practitioners and researchers must always rely on their own experience and knowledge in evaluating and using any information, methods, compounds or experiments described herein. Because of rapid advances in the medical sciences, in particular, independent verification of diagnoses and drug dosages should be made. To the fullest extent of the law, no responsibility is assumed by Elsevier, authors, editors or contributors for any injury and/or damage to persons or property as a matter of products liability, negligence or otherwise, or from any use or operation of any methods, products, instructions, or ideas contained in the material herein.

National Library of Australia Cataloguing-in-Publication Data

A catalogue record for this book is available from the National Library of Australia

Senior Content Strategist: Libby Houston
Content Project Manager: Shubham Dixit
Edited by Jo Crichton
Proofread by Annabel Adair
Cover and Internal design by Lisa Petroff
Index by Innodata Indexing
Typeset by Toppan Best-set Premedia Limited
Printed in China by RR Donnelley Asia

Last digit is the print number: 9 8 7 6 5 4 3 2 1

Contents

Foreword   vii

Preface   viii

About the authors   x

Acknowledgment   x

List of contributors   xi

Chapter 1   Professional practice and portfolios:
                Why is a professional portfolio important?   1

    What is a portfolio?   3

    Forms of portfolios   4

    Portfolios and reflection and lifelong learning   10

    Portfolios and career planning   11

    Conclusion   14

Chapter 2   Portfolio styles and models   15

    What should my portfolio look like?   15

    Privacy, confidentiality and disclosure   19

    Organisation and presentation of portfolios   19

    Steps and responsibilities in portfolio development and use   27

Chapter 3   Reflection and reflective practice   30

    Reflection within professional practice, learning
      and portfolios   30

    Reflective practice   31

    What makes a reflective practitioner?   32

    How does reflection relate to learning?   34

    Tools for reflection   37

    Conclusion   46

Chapter 4   Evidence: What do I have and what do I need?   47

    Where do I start?   48

    What is evidence, and what is its purpose in a
      professional portfolio?   48

	What is quality evidence?	51
	Evidence for portfolios	55
	You have a range of evidence … what next?	57
	Conclusion	60
Chapter 5	**Compiling your portfolio**	**61**
	Deciding on and designing a portfolio framework	62
	Suggested framework for portfolio	62
	Collecting information or evidence	65
	Identifying omissions and generating new evidence	67
	Conclusion	71
Chapter 6	**Portfolio evaluation and assessment**	**72**
	Basic assumptions about assessment	73
	Portfolio approaches and the impact on assessment	73
	Portfolio assessment and evaluation	74
	What is to be assessed?	79
	Conclusion	85
Chapter 7	**Examples of health practitioners' approaches to planning and evaluating CPD**	**88**
	Communicating competence for midwives, registered nurses and enrolled nurses	89
	Communicating competence for midwifery practice	91
	Communicating competence for registered nurse practice	94
	Communicating competence for enrolled nurse practice	100
	Communicating competence for practice in occupational therapy	102
	Communicating competence for practice in paramedicine	106
	Communicating competence for practice in pharmacy	110
	Conclusion	113
References		**114**
Glossary		**118**
Index		**120**

Foreword

The community trusts clinicians and health service organisations to provide safe, high-quality healthcare. Good health outcomes are dependent on the skills and ability of individual clinicians, clinical teams and support staff and the clinical governance, teaching and research capability of health service organisations.

The Australian health system leads in delivery of person-centred care. The fourth edition of *Portfolios for Nursing, Midwifery and other Health Professionals* includes updates that align with person-centred contemporary thinking and practice.

Drs Cusack and Smith are to be congratulated for continuing to evolve this already extensive and comprehensive guide to professional portfolios, and for their significance to the area of professional development more widely.

Importantly, they have kept the elements that made previous instalments such an easy tool to use. The book is practical and jargon-free, and contains many exemplars. There is an emphasis throughout on continuing professional development, and on the importance of reflection and lifelong learning. Multiple options for fulfilling regulatory and professional requirements, and their documentation and recording are also given.

The Australian Commission on Safety and Quality in Health Care (the Commission), is referenced in multiple chapters, and calls on health professionals in the course of the development, review and publication of its multiple and diverse resources for health professionals, managers and consumers of healthcare.

The service provided by people involved in the design, delivery and receiving of healthcare – who participate on consultative committees, working groups and by responding to calls for consultation – contribute enormously to the safety and quality of healthcare in Australia. These individuals, whether they be clinicians, academics, teachers, researchers, administrators, patients or carers, are all involved in the ongoing improvement of healthcare.

Their contributions display critical thinking and analysis. As this book highlights, quality evidence for professional portfolios can take many different forms. The purpose of evidence is simply to provide a foundation for a claim of achievement, and I am delighted to see these contributions also emphasised as another potential building block to that claim.

I highly recommend this book to members of all health professions. There is no doubt in my mind that a continuous focus on professional practice and portfolios directly contributes to Australians receiving safer and high-quality healthcare.

Adjunct Professor Debora Picone AO
Chief Executive Officer, Australian Commission on Safety and Quality in Health Care

Preface

Portfolios are common in university education as a technique for developing reflective analysis skills and demonstrating learning. They are also increasingly used by a range of health professionals as a tool to guide the review of professional practice to direct continuing professional development, learning and career planning, and to communicate professional achievements.

This book will help you to understand the drivers and benefits of portfolios and how to design and evaluate a quality portfolio. Your ability to do this will be assisted by understanding the relationship between professional portfolios and the regulatory requirements of self-declaration and practising in accordance with professional practice standards. The concepts of designing a portfolio for a specific purpose and the use of quality evidence are the central tenets of this book. Where appropriate, supporting materials have been drawn from a range of Australian, New Zealand and international sources. In addition to providing direction on how to design your own professional portfolio, this book contains information about how to evaluate and assess portfolios developed by others.

Because portfolios are widely used in educational and professional settings, this book has relevance to a broad audience, from undergraduate students planning a career as a health professional, through to clinical experts and health administrators. Primarily, however, this book is for individuals intending to develop their own portfolios. In the first instance, readers may wish to peruse this book to gain a basic understanding of portfolios, including how different approaches are used for different purposes, and to gain a sense of the basic process of developing a portfolio. Much of the content that will assist in this is contained in Chapters 1, 2 and 3. Chapters 4 and 5 provide greater detail about understanding your purpose for developing a portfolio, including assembling components and developing an overall argument. Chapter 6 addresses the assessment of portfolios developed by others. This chapter also has relevance to those assembling their own portfolio, for it is through this wider perspective that a complete understanding of a quality portfolio may be gained.

Chapter 7 provides practical examples of differing health practitioners' approaches to using a portfolio to plan their continued professional development.

Each chapter of this book starts with key questions or scenarios that will be explored in the chapter. These are designed to prompt your learning. There is also a glossary of key terms included at the end of the book.

The chapters are organised as follows:

Chapter 1. Professional practice and portfolios: Why is a professional portfolio important?

This chapter assists the reader to understand the concept of portfolios and their use in self-regulation and professional regulation. The contexts of regulation, professional development, learning and career development are used to illustrate the potential for portfolios to guide the review and development of professional practice.

Chapter 2. Portfolio styles and models

Portfolios can be used to direct learning, communicate knowledge and skills and help plan a career. This chapter is designed to enable the reader to appreciate the range of portfolio styles and models, and to identify the need for, and benefits of, specific models to address individual needs. Having examined the purpose for their own portfolio, the reader is introduced to a range of pragmatic issues associated with accumulating and compiling evidence of learning.

Chapter 3. Reflection and reflective practice

The purpose of this chapter is to assist the reader in understanding and applying reflection techniques in professional development, learning and portfolio use. The meanings and uses of the concept of reflection, and their application to the development of portfolios for nurses, midwives and other health professionals, are examined. Specific applications for accomplishing and demonstrating the application and use of reflective skills as a professional achievement are also included.

Chapter 4. Evidence: What do I have and what do I need?

The aim of this chapter is to help the reader to understand the notion of evidence and the types, sources and quality of evidence that will support their knowledge claims. The reader is guided through a process of identifying existing evidence and generating new evidence in support of new knowledge and skills.

Chapter 5. Compiling your portfolio

This chapter helps the reader to develop and assemble a portfolio. The chapter will show the reader how to put together the various parts of a portfolio so that its intent – to produce an account that demonstrates and evaluates progress towards learning and/or professional goals – is achieved.

Chapter 6. Portfolio evaluation and assessment

A quality portfolio is judged through demonstrated proficiency in selecting, structuring and justifying the requisite evidence. This chapter provides an overview of the basic principles of assessment applied to portfolios and is intended not only for the portfolio developer to assess their portfolio development but also as an introduction for those considering a role as an assessor of portfolios for educational and regulatory purposes.

Chapter 7. Examples of health practitioners' approaches to planning and evaluating CPD

This chapter provides practical examples of the approaches used by a range of health practitioners to develop their professional portfolios. Examples have been provided by each of the following: midwife, registered nurse, enrolled nurse, occupational therapist, paramedic and pharmacist.

About the authors

Dr Lynette Cusack RN/midwife, PhD, MHA, BN, DN, MRCN

Dr Cusack is an Associate Professor in the Adelaide Nursing School at the University of Adelaide. Lynette has been involved in a wide range of nursing, midwifery and healthcare policy development, research and education. Contributions include leadership and management, regulation, professional practice development and occupational resilience. Lynette provides practice-based research support to nurses and midwives at a major metropolitan hospital in South Australia. Lynette previously worked in a range of community health settings, including home nursing, community health centres and drug and alcohol services.

Dr Morgan Smith RN, PhD, MEd, BN, Dip App Sc – CHN

Dr Smith is a Senior Lecturer in the Adelaide Nursing School at the University of Adelaide and an Adjunct Lecturer in Nursing at the University of South Australia. Morgan has extensive experience in many areas of both undergraduate and postgraduate nursing education. Her research expertise includes student experiences, engagement and satisfaction with teaching and learning in Bachelor of Nursing programs. She is interested in many areas of nursing practice, primary healthcare and community care, in particular.

Acknowledgment

We would like to thank Kate Andre and Marie Heartfield for their vision, leadership and contribution to the design and content of the earlier editions of the book. We have developed their ideas and hope that we have stayed true to their vision around the purpose, design and application of portfolios for health professionals. We would also like to thank Yvette Salamon for her feedback on chapter 5. It was much appreciated.

List of contributors

Joe Acker PhD (candidate), MA (leadership), GCLTHE, Advanced Care Paramedic
Director of Clinical and Professional Practice, British Columbia Emergency Health Services, Vancouver, BC, Canada; Adjunct Professor, Department of Emergency Medicine, University of British Columbia; Adjunct Senior Lecturer in Paramedicine, Charles Sturt University

Sara Bayes PhD, RN, RM
Associate Professor of Midwifery and Director, Midwifery Studies, School of Nursing and Midwifery, Edith Cowan University, Joondalup, Western Australia

Síobhán Bidgood BA (Hons) (La Trobe), PhD (English)
Psychiatric Enrolled Nurse, SJOG Pinelodge Clinic, Dandenong, Victoria

Lisa Devey BN
Australian Nursing and Midwifery Federation

Susan Gilbert-Hunt M Hlth Sc (Occ Ther), Dip Occ Ther, Cert Teaching Practice Education
Coordinator and Lecturer in the occupational therapy program, School of Health Sciences, University of South Australia

Kearney Gleadhill MPharm, BBiomedSci
Antimicrobial Stewardship/Quality Use of Medicines Pharmacist, Calvary Mater Newcastle Hospital

Professional practice and portfolios: Why is a professional portfolio important?

Introduction

Professional portfolios can assist health practitioners who find themselves in the following situations:

- Your professional registration requires you to make a statement about your competence to practise in line with standards for practice and continuing professional development.
- Your education program or training course has assessments that require portfolio-related activities.
- Your induction into a new job highlights an employment obligation to set and report against individual performance goals.
- You want to develop a career plan.

The above situations are common to most health practitioners at some stage in their careers. They highlight the aim of this book, which is to guide health practitioners in understanding how to develop and present a portfolio that demonstrates their professional efforts, progress, and capacity and capabilities. The book is written for health practitioner students as well as for those already practising in these professions.

This first chapter outlines why it is important to know about professional portfolios and how this record of continuing professional development can be useful in providing information when planning a career change or submitting a job application, or in order to meet the requirements of others, such as:

- *Health practitioner regulatory authorities:* for purposes of initial registration or renewal of registration.
- *Educational providers:* to pass a course or program, or to apply for recognition of prior learning.
- *Employers;* to gain employment or promotion.
- *Professional organisations:* for accreditation and/or credential purposes.

As health practitioners, we use our knowledge, experience and evidence to improve the health experiences of the people in our care. Portfolios provide a way to present that knowledge and evidence in a format that communicates to others our learning and development, as well as our current level of achievement, capability and competency.

An individual creating a professional portfolio needs to examine their current practice against appropriate expectations, role or position descriptions or standards (be they personal or professional). This process will highlight potential areas for improvement and in doing so inform a learning or career plan for continuing professional development. Different or higher standards of practice open the way for new opportunities, as well as professional and career development.

The obligations placed on health practitioners are complex. As discussed in more detail later in this chapter, health practitioners have legal and moral obligations both as members of their professions and as individuals. These obligations also extend to employers. The external pressures to demonstrate the appropriateness of their clinical and professional decisions have also increased considerably. Since October 2004, when the World Health Organization launched the World Alliance for Patient Safety, most countries, including Australia, have established a range of national healthcare safety and quality mechanisms with the clear message that professional competence and ongoing education impact directly on patient safety (Australian Commission on Safety and Quality in Health Care 2011). The demands on health systems and services directly impact on the health workforce and its training and service delivery.

In Australia, health consumers expect clinicians to assist them to be better informed, manage their health where possible, and provide prompt and appropriate individualised help if necessary (Taylor & Hill 2014). The rise of the health consumer movement, particularly in the last decade or so, means that patients and their carers now have a justifiable and much more noticeable voice, along with increasing expectations about healthcare and what clinicians can offer (Australian Commission on Safety and Quality in Health Care 2011). Unfortunately, increased expectations of what could be provided will not always translate to what can or must be provided.

An implication of this situation for healthcare students and practitioners is the clear need for skills in understanding, generating and using evidence that communicates how their practice meets the necessary standards of professional responsibility and accountability. This book will examine the different forms that such evidence can take, as well as the skills (such as reflection) that are necessary in producing the evidence and the arguments for continuing professional development.

Health practitioners have significant responsibilities in providing health interventions and protecting patients from the effects of illness, disability and infirmity. A significant and continuing challenge for all healthcare practitioners is to stay informed about the knowledge developments and recommended practice changes that are relevant to their field and role. This responsibility becomes increasingly important the more complex healthcare becomes. Factors affecting the complexity of healthcare include an ageing population, challenges in the management of chronic disease and increasing shifts to primary healthcare, relatively rapid changes in client conditions and expectations, developments in pharmacology and the use of technology, and changes in health systems and practitioner roles.

All healthcare practitioners have an obligation to improve the quality of client care and to manage threats to client safety. The best-available evidence is necessary as a foundation for all health practitioner actions. The only effective way to manage these expectations is to be continuously learning and engaging with the healthcare and professional agendas that affect our practice. Health practitioners in Australia and New Zealand are required to demonstrate their continuing professional development and engagement as a condition of their registration to practise. Portfolios have a long and reliable history as a useful way to demonstrate purposeful learning and engagement with practice and, therefore, progressive skill development and capacity building.

SUMMARY POINTS

- The purpose of this book is to provide a depth of understanding about why portfolios can support nurses, midwives and other health practitioners to develop and extend their practice and careers.
- All health practitioners in Australia and New Zealand have legal and moral obligations to demonstrate understanding and evidence of their continuing level of competency to practise.
- Engagement with their profession and ongoing development of their professional capacity are conditions of registration for all health practitioners.

As a first step in learning about portfolios and gaining the confidence to create one, the following discussion outlines the various types of portfolios and the main reasons for their use.

What is a portfolio?

The word 'portfolio' is used in various ways, depending on the context of use. In a political or organisational sense, a portfolio shows an allocation of responsibilities. In education, a portfolio is usually a collection of information that informs the demonstration of learning that has occurred for an individual in a specific course or program of studies. A professional portfolio is structured evidence demonstrating that an individual is meeting their profession's standards for practice, including an indication of the professional's vision of future growth and capacity building. It shows the individual's continuing professional development activities and experiences, competencies, and professional achievements and goals. It is both a source of detail and a means by which the portfolio author or developer acquires and develops skills in reflective analysis and communication.

A portfolio is more than a collection of documents, certificates, photographs and other artefacts collected over a working life. It takes its shape as a professional portfolio through the reflections and connections that are built by the portfolio author or developer. Connections are the links between the actual experiences, practices, thoughts and ideas, and the relevant or necessary frameworks, standards, tools or expectations of the individual nurse or midwife and their profession. These connections are created and described by the individual portfolio author most commonly through reflective thinking and analysis. The frameworks, standards, tools or expectations that might shape a portfolio could be standards for registration, practice or education; specialty, competency or continuing professional development standards as endorsed in Australia by the National Boards that are part of the National Registration and Accreditation Scheme (Australian Health Practitioner Regulation Agency 2019a); or even national safety and quality standards (Australian Commission on Safety and Quality in Health Care 2012). For a student, the framework guiding the aim and structure of a portfolio may be directed by the requirements of a particular course assignment.

The reflective process of examining current practice across personal, professional, organisational, regulatory, social and technological dimensions provides the insights needed to record past professional development and the focus for continued development. The outcomes of this process provide a basis from which to demonstrate the capacity to provide quality and safe care, and to contribute competently to your relevant health profession and organisation.

A portfolio demonstrates thinking and reasoning, and in this sense it is an argument in that it gives reasons, or cites evidence, in support of an idea, action or theory in an attempt to get others to share a point of view. An argument is identifiable by a logical or quasi-logical sequence of ideas supported by evidence (Andrews 2010) with the important addition of a clear outcome or conclusion.

An effective professional portfolio not only includes descriptions of experiences and practice but links this to the relevant health professional knowledge and debate to justify the level of expertise or learning that has been achieved. The portfolio outlines why the claim is legitimate and can be accepted as valid in meeting the required expectations. This type of portfolio applies health professional knowledge to the clinical and other practice of the individual in their particular context or circumstances.

Variations on what a portfolio looks like, how it is used or why it is needed are all influenced by who is seeking what information and for what purpose. Healthcare is based on the principle of evidence for practice. Implementing evidence entails asking an answerable question in a particular situation, acquiring the best relevant evidence, appraising that evidence critically, then integrating it into decision-making in a way that accords with the client's preference (Brown et al. 2010). So, in the context of a professional portfolio, 'evidence' means the information or verification that may be interpreted as support for your claims. Evidence may be produced by others (such as a certificate of achievement) or by the individual (such as through reflective thinking). Evidence will be discussed in more detail in Chapter 3.

The evidence necessary to acquire and demonstrate expertise or learning is complex, takes time to put together, and varies depending on practice context, education and experience. A professional portfolio, in whatever format, includes a range of documents, such as certificates of attendance at continuing professional development (CPD) events and courses, linked through processes of reflective analysis to demonstrate past and current achievements with future-oriented goals for competent health professional practice.

Forms of portfolios

Portfolios can take many forms. Compilations of hard copy documents related to your working life are probably the most familiar portfolio format. However, developments in knowledge, information and learning

---

SUMMARY POINTS

- A professional portfolio is a collection of resources and a means by which to develop skills in reflective analysis and communication.
- Portfolios help to demonstrate and support the following:
  - individual reflective thinking and writing processes
  - employment, education, and professional and personal development
  - performance based on analysis of previous and current practice
  - competence based on analysis of previous and current knowledge, skills and experiences
  - application of knowledge to practice through an understanding of how context may shape competency and practice
  - learning based on knowledge acquisition and skill development
  - future goals and career direction based on consideration and analysis of the previous two points.

ACTIVITY: PROFESSIONAL ROLES

As a first step in building a portfolio, write a brief description about your current role, including responsibilities, accountabilities and challenges as well as positive affirmations you have received. The purpose of this is to provide a background to reflect upon as you start to compile your portfolio, which is discussed in detail in Chapter 5.

It is a good idea to keep this description accessible so that you can review and build on it as your portfolio develops.

technologies have prompted the emergence of digital or electronic portfolios that support reflective processes and professional collaborations. As discussed in greater detail in Chapter 2, there are various software programs available to assist in producing these electronic collections of scanned documents or files.

Electronic portfolios enable you to format and arrange the different pieces of evidence or portfolio items to produce different versions of your portfolio, depending on its intended purpose and the specific requirements of the portfolio reader. For example, the portfolio may be intended only for personal use or for preparing assignments, or it may be submitted in response to a professional audit of your continued professional development by the relevant health practitioner regulator.

As Fig. 1.1 shows, at the base level a portfolio can provide a repository of evidence of your professional practice, including résumés, education and registration certificates, employment records, performance appraisals,

references, letters, and other related documents such as records of committee membership or volunteer activities. The final portfolio, however, needs to be developed in a manner that reflects both an understanding of, and adherence to, professional standards. Personal reflective statements can trace the processes that have occurred in achieving this, including professional engagement, accessing and using evidence to enhance practice, and identifying areas of future development. These reflective and critical accounts of practice or learning enable you, as the portfolio author, to demonstrate deep learning about complex issues. Examples of these types of statements would be experiences and improvements in ethical understanding or clinical decision-making, which can be difficult to demonstrate in other ways. This type of evidence can assist the portfolio reader, such as your employer or lecturer, to assess shifts or developments in your learning and levels of competence.

Portfolios will contain multiple documents, including both official and personal papers, some of which may remain confidential to the author and must not be shared with others. Disclosure, privacy legislation and self-protection are addressed in more detail in Chapter 2, along with suggested portfolio structures. An example of a specific structure would be where professional standards or competencies are used as headings, with evidence that demonstrates the levels of knowledge, skill and performance.

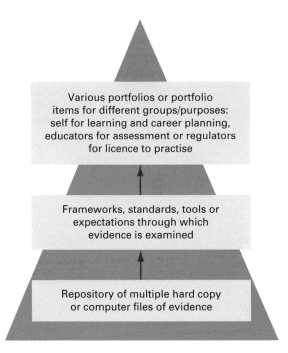

Figure 1.1 Portfolio components

Various portfolios or portfolio items for different groups/purposes: self for learning and career planning, educators for assessment or regulators for licence to practise

Frameworks, standards, tools or expectations through which evidence is examined

Repository of multiple hard copy or computer files of evidence

SUMMARY POINTS

- A professional portfolio is more than a résumé or curriculum vitae. It is more than a collection of education and registration certificates, employment details, log of events, or practice- or learning-related documents.
- A professional portfolio is a broad and structured mix of different resources. These resources are collected or produced through a career-long process of continuous professional development and result in various portfolio items or products that can be used for different purposes.

Regulation of professional practice and the requirement for communicating competence through a professional portfolio

The following discussion examines some issues that health practitioners must consider when constructing a professional portfolio.

Health practitioners are subject to a range of forms of regulation. Regulation for the protection of the public requires prescribing and enforcing standards and codes of practice that are relevant to the capabilities for safe and effective practice (Benton et al. 2015). The various regulatory frameworks for each health profession set out the different requirements for practice through both legislative and non-legal processes. These different types of regulation are discussed next, starting with the statutory regulation of health practitioners.

In Australia, the National Registration and Accreditation Scheme was established in 2010 under the *Health Practitioner Regulation National Law Act 2009* ('National Law') in each state and territory. The Australian Health Practitioner Regulation Agency (AHPRA) currently partners with 15 National Boards that regulate health professions in the public interest (Australian Health Practitioner Regulation Agency 2019b). The health professions that are currently regulated in Australia are: Aboriginal and Torres Strait Islander practitioners, chiropractors, dentists (with dental hygienists, dental prosthetists and dental therapists), medical practitioners, medical radiation practitioners, nurses, midwives, occupational therapists, optometrists, osteopaths, pharmacists, physiotherapists, podiatrists, psychologists and paramedics (Australian Health Practitioner Regulation Agency 2019b).

The National Law makes specific reference to registration standards, accreditation, notifications and conduct, health and performance, and privacy and information sharing.

In New Zealand, there are 22 health professions regulated by specified authorities under the *Health Practitioners Competence Assurance Act 2003*. This Act requires health practitioners to demonstrate their competence to practise and their professional education

in new skills and technologies. The protected nursing and midwifery titles are the same for New Zealand and Australia: registered nurse, midwife, enrolled nurse and nurse practitioner.

Portfolios and regulation requirement for continuing professional development

All of the Australian National Boards have a specific continuing professional development standard that is required to be met by those individuals registered with that National Board. These standards specify the requirements that the registered health practitioner must meet to maintain their licence to practise. Continuing professional development is made up of the actions taken by the registered health practitioner to develop the personal and professional qualities that are necessary to their professional lives. This includes maintaining, improving, and extending or expanding their knowledge, expertise and competence.

Each continuing professional development standard includes any specific requirements for the professional. This may include the requirement for a learning plan, the number of hours (or credits or points) that need to be spent on learning activities, and a report on the professional development activities undertaken that includes reflection on their value. See Chapter 7 for an example of how different health practitioners interpret their continuing professional development requirements. Continuing professional development records, such as a portfolio, need to demonstrate that the health practitioner has:

- evaluated their practice against the competency or professional practice standards, relevant to their context of practice, to identify and prioritise their learning needs
- developed a learning plan based on identified learning needs
- participated in effective learning activities relevant to their learning needs
- reflected on the value of the learning activities or the effect of participation on their practice.

To be part of a regulated profession requires health practitioners to fully understand their responsibility and accountability for standards of practice and competence. Health practitioner regulatory authorities provide, under legislation, various codes, guidelines, standards and competency statements to protect the public and to support health practitioners to practise safely and ethically. As mentioned earlier, these documents as well as any others related to your employment, are useful in guiding the development of a learning plan recorded within a portfolio.

Key resources are provided here, to assist you to stay informed about your professional obligations. Such understanding may guide your future-learning plan and be captured within a portfolio.

RESOURCES

Useful websites for understanding health practitioner regulation in Australia and New Zealand include the following:

1 The Australian Health Practitioner Regulation Agency (www.ahpra.gov.au) regulates the Australian health workforce through the following National Boards:
   - Aboriginal and Torres Strait Islander Health Practice Board of Australia
   - Chinese Medicine Board of Australia
   - Chiropractic Board of Australia
   - Dental Board of Australia
   - Medical Board of Australia
   - Medical Radiation Practice Board of Australia
   - Nursing and Midwifery Board of Australia
   - Occupational Therapy Board of Australia
   - Optometry Board of Australia
   - Osteopathy Board of Australia
   - Paramedicine Board of Australia
   - Pharmacy Board of Australia
   - Physiotherapy Board of Australia
   - Podiatry Board of Australia
   - Psychology Board of Australia.

2 The New Zealand Ministry of Health (www.health.govt.nz/our-work/regulation-health-and-disability -system/health-practitioners-competence-assurance-act/responsible-authorities-under-act) regulates its health workforce through the following regulatory authorities:
   - Chiropractic Board
   - Dental Council (covering dentistry, dental hygiene, clinical dental technology, dental technology and dental therapy)
   - Dietitians Board
   - Medical Council
   - Medical Radiation Technologists Board
   - Medical Sciences Council of New Zealand (medical laboratory science and anaesthetic technology)

- Midwifery Council
- Nursing Council
- Occupational Therapy Board
- Optometrists and Dispensing Opticians Board
- Osteopathic Council
- Pharmacy Council
- Physiotherapy Board
- Podiatrists Board
- Psychologists Board
- Psychotherapists Board.

Other regulation requirements for consideration when building a portfolio

As well as the health practitioner regulation Acts, there are other laws in the Australian states and territories that specify responsibilities for health practitioners. Examples of these are laws concerning therapeutic or controlled substances, mental health, aged care, immunisation and child/elder abuse.

Processes other than laws that regulate the way health practitioners practise include various health industry standards and accreditation processes, such as those developed to guide health and social care in particular contexts (e.g. quality and safety, and aged care). The provision of healthcare services at the organisational level is also governed (i.e. regulated) through numerous levels and mechanisms, which may be linked to funding or accreditation to provide services. Professional organisations such as colleges and special interest groups also play a role in shaping the practice of individuals and the professions through various lobbying, policy, guideline and standards development activities. Can you name the professional organisation or college for your discipline? In nursing, an alliance of over 56 national nursing and midwifery specialty organisations aims to advance the nursing profession to improve healthcare (Coalition of National Nursing and Midwifery Organisations 2015). Many of these organisations produce competency or practice standards for the practitioners in those fields (see Table 1.1 overleaf). The portfolio is an excellent location to record the identified competencies or practice standards that can be used to guide the development of a learning plan or career pathway if you are contemplating change to your context of practice.

Employing organisations regulate health practitioners through organisational standards and the various industrial awards and agreements that specify roles and employment conditions, such as salary and leave entitlements. These documents, relevant to your context of practice and professional development, should also be referred to in your portfolio because this communicates your broader understanding of the various key legislative and policy documents that shape your professional responsibilities and accountabilities.

SUMMARY POINTS

- It is necessary for all regulated health practitioners to apply the standards endorsed by their regulating body, relevant to context of practice.
- It is useful to keep a portfolio, because you can communicate your understanding of the professional groups and individual health practitioners' mandatory and voluntary professional obligations.
- Portfolios provide a useful means to track changes in practice and performance as healthcare becomes increasingly complex and open to scrutiny through governance and audits of standards of care.

TABLE 1.1

Members of the Australian Coalition of National Nursing and Midwifery Organisations

- Audiometry Nurses Association of Australia (ANAA)
- Australasian Cardiovascular Nursing College (ACNC)
- Australasian College for Infection Prevention and Control
- Australasian Hepatology Association
- Australasian Neuroscience Nurses' Association
- Australasian Rehabilitation Nurses' Association Inc. (ARNA)
- Australasian Sexual Health and HIV Nurses Association
- Australian Association of Stomal Therapy Nurses Inc.
- Australian Association of Nurse Surgical Assistants
- Australian College of Children and Young People's Nurses
- Australian College of Critical Care Nurses (ACCCN)
- Australian College of Holistic Nurses Inc. (ACHN)
- Australian College of Mental Health Nurses Inc. (ACMHN)
- Australian College of Midwives (ACM)
- Australian College of Neonatal Nurses (ACNN)
- Australian College of Nurse Practitioners (ACNP)
- Australian College of Nursing (ACN)
- Australian College of Perioperative Nurses (ACORN)
- Australian Day Surgery Nurses Association (ADSNA)
- Australian Dermatology Nurses Association
- Australian Diabetes Educators Association (ADEA)
- Australian Faith Community Nurses Association
- Australian Forensic Nurses Association
- Australian and New Zealand Orthopaedic Nurses Association
- Australian and New Zealand Society for Vascular Nurses (ANZSVN)
- Australian and New Zealand Urological Nurses Society (ANZUNS)
- Australian Nurse Teachers' Society
- Australian Nursing and Midwifery Federation (ANMF)
- Australian Ophthalmic Nurses Association National Council (AONANC)
- Australian Primary Health Care Nurses Association
- Australian Student and Novice Nurse Association (ASANNA)
- Australian Women's Health Nurse Association Inc.
- Cancer Nurses Society of Australia
- College of Emergency Nursing Australia
- Congress of Aboriginal and Torres Strait Islander Nurses (CATSIN)
- Continence Nurses Society Australia (CoNSA)
- Council of Deans of Nursing and Midwifery (Australia & New Zealand)
- CRANAplus
- Discharge Planning Association
- Drug and Alcohol Nurses of Australasia (Inc.) (DANA)
- Endocrine Nurses Society of Australasia
- Flight Nurses Australia Inc.
- Gastroenterological Nurses College of Australia (GENCA)
- Hyperbaric Technicians and Nurses Association
- Maternal Child & Family Health Nurses of Australia (MCFHNA)
- Medical Imaging Nurses Association (MINA)
- National Enrolled Nurses Association of Australia (NENA)
- Nursing Informatics Australia (NIA)
- Otorhinolaryngology, Head & Neck Nurses Group Inc.
- Palliative Care Nurses Australia
- Psychogeriatric Nurses Association Australia Inc. (PGNA)
- Renal Society of Australasia
- Thoracic Society of Australia and New Zealand
- Transplant Nurses Association
- Wounds Australia

ACTIVITY: COMMENCING YOUR PORTFOLIO

Completing the following questions and activities will help you to understand the links between keeping a professional portfolio and evidence of healthcare knowledge and skill development.

1 Who authorises or regulates your ability to practise as a registered health professional?

2 Who assesses your learning and development, either as a student or in your employment position?

3 What do these individuals or organisations require as evidence of your ability to do your job successfully or to demonstrate learning?

4 Do they specify a template or format in which this information needs to be presented (such as annual performance reviews)? *Tip:* A number of the National Boards provide quite detailed guidelines about what is involved in meeting their continuing professional development standards. These resources may be useful for other health practitioners if they require some guidance on developing a template for their portfolio.

5 Do they provide guidelines about the types, volumes or forms of evidence they require?

In answering these questions, it will be useful to use the internet to search for the specific codes, standards or guidelines that are used to regulate your practice. It is a good idea to know who produces or endorses these standards and how they are used to regulate your practice. They will be discussed in greater detail in subsequent chapters.

6 As a further activity, you might expand your information search strategies to compare the standards for practice for different professions. For example, if you are a nurse or nursing student, you may find it useful to compare the standards for practice for the registered nurse with those of the enrolled nurse or nurse practitioner.

7 Go to the AHPRA or relevant country health practitioner regulation authority website and view the relevant accreditation and registration standards for your health profession. If you are undertaking entry-to-practice education, this site will list for you the standards you need to meet in order to register when your studies are completed.

Portfolios and reflection and lifelong learning

Most of us accept that change is constant and that we must learn the skills necessary to engage with what work and life have to offer. The concept of adult learning suggests that one of the reasons adults are motivated to learn is because they understand that learning is necessary to be able to perform in their professional or work roles (Knowles et al. 2015). There are also links between the social, technical and personal dimensions of our lives that impact not only on our individual professional growth and development but also on the remaking and changing of professional practice (Chertoff et al. 2016, Laux & Stoten 2016). Technology plays a key part in all aspects of our professional and personal lives and is particularly relevant with the growth in e-portfolios or similar platforms that allow professional online interactions.

Lifelong learning skills equip health practitioners to manage the significant responsibilities of their roles. Lifelong learning skills include being:

* information literate, which means being able to locate, evaluate, manage and use information in a range of contexts

- an effective communicator, which means being competent in the required level of reading, writing, speaking and listening
- self-aware, which means being able to understand and make maximum benefit of personal strengths and accept personal limitations
- contextually aware, which means being able to identify and find ways to manage the social, political, cultural and environmental influences on practice.

So, if we accept learning as a continuous part of professional practice, then it is important also to understand that learning is more than just remembering new information. We move from superficial or surface knowledge to a deeper understanding through complex psychological, social and emotional learning processes. Reflective thinking is one example of these processes (Chertoff et al. 2016). Reflection is an important process in portfolio development. It is the examination or exploration of experiences with the aim of generating new understandings and appreciation (Chertoff et al. 2016).

Reflection has a long history in education programs for nursing, midwifery and other health professions (Chertoff et al. 2016, Clouder & Sellars 2004, Mills 2009). This is because it is seen as a way to bring together knowledge and theory with practice or clinical actions. Knowledge is developed through rational processes of understanding scientific and theoretical information. However, we know that other types of knowledge come from other sources, and that the challenge for practice-based knowledge comes from linking theory, personal interpretation, experience and culture (Egan & Testa 2010, p. 153).

Reflective processes are attributed with making more apparent or obvious the knowledge and learning that occurs in practice (Bolton 2005). Skills in reflection help to differentiate between the facts that we know and how we interpret them, and then how we might use this knowledge and interpretation in practice (Hull et al. 2005). A professional portfolio can be used to communicate the bringing together of critical thinking, analysis, synthesis and evaluation of learning from practice and peers in order to generate new learning and knowledge about practice (Clouder & Sellars 2004).

> **SUMMARY POINTS**
>
> - Reflection is an important process in portfolio development.
> - Lifelong learning involves both informal and formal learning and requires self-motivation to participate in learning to do an existing job, develop new ways of doing a job or retrain for a new job.
> - Practice-based knowledge is developed by reflective thinking – that is, thinking through and developing links between theory, personal interpretation, experience and culture. Having reflective thinking and analysis skills helps nurses, midwives and other health practitioners to counteract the complexity of the health system, where often there are no prescribed right or wrong answers.

Portfolios and career planning

While much of the previous discussion has been about looking back over practice to develop a statement about competency for current practice, portfolios also have a major function in assisting you to look forward and develop a career plan (Laux & Stoten 2016).

Career planning is not just about a series of jobs. A career is about purposefully linking your mix of work, learning and life (MCEECDYA 2010). Portfolios assist health practitioners with career planning.

For the majority of health practitioners who work in the employment of others, the relationship with their organisation is an important consideration. While the focus of this relationship is mostly about performance, the role of organisations in career development has also changed. Employment is only one of a range of ways in which organisations help to shape an individual's career. Some other ways are by providing education, training and credentialling, and funding career development opportunities and activities.

Career planning for health practitioners needs to consider projected changes in healthcare, such as the impact of technology and ageing populations and shifts towards interdisciplinary and home-based healthcare. These changes generate opportunities for health practitioners to be actively responsible for their futures. An example might be to think more broadly about identifying the education programs that are best suited to accommodate trends in health service delivery. Examples of such trends relevant to health practitioners are the growth in public and population health programs, and in quality improvement and risk management.

Health professionals need to be career-resilient by being flexible and adaptable. The following discussion examines how portfolios can assist in career planning.

Career-planning steps

Portfolios can be used to capture key career-planning steps to support moving purposefully forward. Self-awareness is a key part of ongoing professional development, and career planning and development. Career development is the term that best describes a complex process of managing life, learning and work over the lifespan (MCEECDYA 2010). Career planning allows you to capitalise on your motivation and make informed decisions (or to overcome poor motivation or continued indecision) and focus your efforts towards purposefully set career goals.

As previously discussed, portfolios provide a way for you to review, refine, evaluate and re-evaluate both your current situation and your goals and progress plans for the future. Goal-setting can be motivating in achieving short- and long-term goals. Goals need to be linked by an overarching vision of what you want to achieve in your working life and the values, beliefs, skills and work interests that are rewarding to you. It is important for health practitioners to set goals to ensure that they plan not only their future employment but also their career pathways; they also need contingency plans in case their goals are not met. Understanding, predicting and attending to changing healthcare deliveries will further enhance the likelihood of meeting your personal goals.

Portfolios offer a place in which to store all the information relevant to your career. The portfolio development process outlined in this book involves self-reflection and evaluation of your knowledge, skills, current practice and experiences, as well as analysis of other perspectives, the available evidence and generated new evidence. This information is supplemented with statements about how to plan and record the achievement of learning knowledge and skills. In this way, portfolios help describe your professional strengths and limitations, and can be used as a marketing and self-promotional tool, being submitted during the application process and referred to during job interviews. Portfolios also provide a career development plan that overrides daily work activities and pressures. It can focus what you do at work and help you to manage workplace stresses and demands and prepare yourself for change.

Portfolios provide a basis for better understanding your preferences and skills in ways that show your suitability for certain professional contexts or areas of work. By identifying trends in performance evaluations or other forms of feedback, a professional portfolio can act as a map to the things that need to be done to progress your career decisions and plans. A portfolio may highlight areas that can be raised in performance review sessions for future development. To achieve this, portfolios need to be examined as an entire collection of experiences. This collection is then organised not only according to competencies but also based on past achievements and strategic plans that address personal or organisational goals. In order to use a portfolio for career planning, the details need to be organised with attention to your strengths, limitations and preferences, as well as your achievements, experiences and expertise in areas of practice.

Career planning using a portfolio involves thinking beyond your current situation. Your aims are to think about what goals, roles or positions you want to achieve, what actions you need to take and with what resources, and, lastly, how you will know when you have reached or achieved your goals. Career planning requires self- and peer assessment, research into your area of work, decision-making and goal-setting, regular reviews of résumés and periodic reviews of job opportunities. With an e-portfolio, this can be achieved in collaboration with your peers, supervisors or mentors via invited feedback. Chapter 2 will provide further details on how this might be achieved.

RESOURCES

Individual discipline groups have devised resources to assist in career planning. While it is important to be familiar with those associated with your own discipline, given the broad principles that will apply to all of us, you might also find it useful to review others as well.

There are many career counselling resources and services available through internet searches, or through events such as open days and seminars provided by universities or professional organisations. Most universities provide generic career-planning resources and services for new applicants or graduates. These may be available online or as individual counselling for students. The websites of government health, employment and education departments, and some professional organisations, often include career-planning tools and information. A career self-assessment tool can be useful for students and graduates to help develop or reassess career goals and identify the actions necessary to achieve these goals. One such resource is the *Your Career and You* booklet (Graduate Careers Australia).

National and international professional organisations and government health department websites are useful places to visit to keep track of developments in healthcare and associated employment opportunities. Reading employment advertisements on a regular basis will also provide you with insight into the types of positions that are available and the associated requirements, remuneration and benefits. You will probably note, for example, the increase in nursing positions in quality and risk management, aged and community care, and general practice.

It is a good idea to discuss your career plans with others to get new information or ideas worth considering. This may also highlight other ideas or perspectives you had not thought about. Engagement with professional colleagues and networks is important. Mentors, colleagues, family, friends and supervisors can provide valuable professional guidance. Usually, mentoring involves an ongoing professional relationship often within the employing organisation (Irby 2012).

A mentor is not the same as a preceptor or supervisor, who is focused on what you have to do in your job. There are many online resources about mentoring, but, because mentoring is about interaction with others, a better source may be to find the nursing and midwifery organisations that have links to mentoring opportunities. Alternatively, just getting out and networking with members of your profession may assist you in meeting like-minded, willing, experienced and appropriate people to help you develop your potential.

ACTIVITY: IDENTIFYING EXISTING PORTFOLIO INFORMATION AND EVIDENCE

Make a list of the documents you already have that relate to either your health practitioner studies or employment. If these are in hard copy form, consider scanning them to start building your online portfolio.

Do these documents show any broader professional or inter-professional engagement?

Are you a member of, or have you visited the website for, the peak body for your discipline or profession?

SUMMARY POINTS

- People play a significant part in the construction and development of their own careers. However, career planning is more than setting individual goals.
- Active engagement with professional networks and mentors is important for work satisfaction and quality practice outcomes.
- Reflection on individual professional practice and the broader healthcare contexts prompts the identification of current and future learning needs that can inform the ways forward for career planning and development.
- Developing a professional portfolio helps you to learn a process for reviewing and re-evaluating your goals and plans for the future, as well as providing a place to manage this information.

Conclusion

In this chapter, portfolios have been presented as part of professional practice – that is, they are linked to understanding the individual and collective obligations for regulated practice. Health practitioners enter their professional practice following successful completion of specific tertiary or vocational qualifications. This education is designed to equip them with the skills for continued learning, and employers and regulatory authorities will require individual practitioners to continue this learning after entry to practice in order to achieve a quality health service. This responsibility includes the need to keep sufficient quality evidence of practice and performance. The National Boards' requirements for continuing professional development illustrate how this ongoing learning is a lifelong responsibility for continuing competence for professional practice.

This chapter has focused on portfolios for professional practice, while also recognising that portfolios have a place in assessment of learning as part of educational programs, organisational performance reviews and individual career plans. The focus on key developments in the regulation of health practitioners has set the scene for understanding that a professional portfolio is more than a means of collecting and reflecting on evidence of learning or practice. It is a way to communicate, showcase and improve skilled healthcare practice with the collective aim of improving the quality of the health system by growing the intellectual capital.

Portfolio styles and models

Introduction

- Where do you start in designing your portfolio?
- What are the necessary and optional parts?
- What are the benefits and challenges of using an electronic platform to develop and display your portfolio?
- What are the challenges and potential risks in using electronic portfolios?

Moving on from understanding why it is necessary or useful to develop a professional portfolio, this chapter focuses on the variety of styles and models of portfolios as well as the purposes for which they might be used.

Searching the word 'portfolio' on the internet will expose the many uses of this term, as well as numerous formats, guides, templates and products. A range of these are available from a variety of educational, commercial, regulatory and employment sources. Some guides are for purchase or are distributed as part of professional memberships, while others are available for free. Many of them are similar in design, with guidelines on how to bring together your career goals with your record of continuing professional development. This chapter will demonstrate how the main issue is not really which style you use to develop a professional portfolio; rather, it is how your format supports your intended portfolio use.

An overview of portfolio styles and features is followed by exercises for you to work through to help you meet the needs of your portfolio readership. The chapter ends with a detailed examination of electronic forms of portfolios, or e-portfolios.

What should my portfolio look like?

As mentioned in Chapter 1, most people start their 'portfolio journey' as a response to the expectations or requirements of an external group such as a university course, employer or regulatory authority. Alternatively, you may put together a portfolio because you need evidence of job performance, or because you are applying for a promotion or a new job. The purpose of different portfolios will vary, and it is important to think about your specific aim and other possible uses before choosing

the design for your portfolio. Through understanding the purpose of your first portfolio, and then through ongoing use, you will come to value the suitability of some approaches over others. For example, you may be a confident and regular computer user, so the idea of an electronic portfolio is immediately appealing. Also, your initial experiences in bringing together or creating relevant information (evidence) will introduce you to deciding how to tag or code it for possible future use.

Portfolio models

There are as many different formats of portfolios as there are purposes. Most health practitioner portfolios are personal collections of employer- or educator-provided and self-constructed materials about education and practice, with some professional observations or reports on your practice by others. This chapter will extend your understanding of physical forms by introducing electronic or digital portfolios.

Portfolio models have been given names such as 'shopping trolley', 'toast rack', 'spinal column' and 'cake mix' (Jasper et al. 2013) in an attempt to illustrate the differences in portfolio structures. While all such models had their uses in career planning, educational assessment or performance evaluation, most had limitations. These included an overreliance on self-reported data and a lack of sufficient linking and explanation of evidence – what we refer to as development of an argument that demonstrates achievement. This also made portfolios very difficult to assess with any accuracy, as reflected in the literature about assessing continuing competency (Fricke 2015). In most models, portfolios include both evidence and a rationale in support of the evidence.

Portfolios may be primarily about learning, showcasing achievement or both. Portfolios may have two interconnected spaces and functions; one is a workspace where learning and development occurs, and the other is a showcase where outcomes are demonstrated (Barrett 2010). Interconnection is not essential and may be potentially problematic for reasons that will be explored shortly. The principles are relevant to paper-based or e-portfolios.

The 'portfolio as a learning workspace', is the process-focused activity of generating a repository of artefacts and personal reflections. Generally, material is generated and stored chronologically with the main aim being to reflect upon and enhance personal learning. The reflection is directed at a specific and recent experience or event, with the focus being, 'What and how can I learn from this?' (Barrett 2010). If you read more widely about portfolios, you will find that many texts written from an educational perspective will focus on this 'learning through reflection' aspect of portfolios. Privacy and confidentiality are important when creating portfolios as a learning space. Reflections on practice can involve highly sensitive information and it is important such reflections, even where confidentiality and privacy is maintained, are securely stored.

The 'portfolio as showcase' is a product that displays personal professional accountability by substantiating an argument of competence through the provision of workplace evidence. Individuals will have multiple versions of these 'achievement portfolios' that address different criteria depending on the job, promotion or other intended use. These versions will often draw on the same evidence, but will be structured to address the needs of the new audience. In electronic form, these audiences can access specific portfolios through varied online permissions. The 'achievement showcase' portfolio is for external audiences and is organised thematically around achievement criteria, such as professional standards or institutional goals. Reflection is still important in this form of portfolio, but it is more focused on understanding past achievements to inform future plans (Barrett 2010). An achievement showcase should ensure confidentiality of information relating to others. There is a range of literature about achievement or product-oriented portfolios, particularly by organisations associated with professional accountability.

The components of and interactions between these two portfolio approaches are explained further in the following chapters of this book.

What is an e-portfolio?

In its most basic form, an e-portfolio is an electronic way to collate, structure, store, format, present and reconfigure materials or artefacts, including text, images, video and sound, in a manner that shows an individual's 'skills, knowledge, experiences and processes through which one

develops personally and professionally, over an extended period of time' (Hallam et al. 2010, p. 11). Initially, e-portfolios were merely used to transfer text and images into electronic form, similar to that of an electronic curriculum vitae. There are instances where there has been little progress beyond this, such that users compile their paper-based achievement records and convert these to electronic portable document format (PDF) files to enable them to submit the portfolio via an online portal. This in itself is an advanced form of paper-based portfolios, as the original document remains with the individual and, depending on computer access, the submission process can be convenient and time efficient. This approach serves many institutions well, for having applicants submit documentary evidence in electronic form provides the convenience of not having to sort the post, file the various documents and maintain the paper records. However, as this chapter details, e-portfolios can also include additional supports designed to assist with the development of artefacts, enhance reflective processes, extend learning and achievements via selective and specific interaction with others, store and retrieve artefacts, and produce quality portfolio displays that depict the complexity of achievements through the inclusion of audio and visual images. A national audit found a high level of interest and activity related to e-portfolios in the Australian higher education and vocational education and training sector (Hallam & Creagh 2010).

Who is the intended audience for my portfolio?

Although portfolios are likely to contain sections that are private and not designed to be read by others, most complete portfolios are written for specific readers. Knowing who the readers of your portfolio will be, and what their expectations are, is important in ensuring your portfolio is successful in communicating your intended message. In most cases, the intended audience for a completed portfolio is university lecturers, line managers, staff development officers or professional regulatory assessors. Understanding the role of these people in reading and reviewing your portfolio, and being aware of the criteria they will use in evaluating it, can be a real advantage in structuring and designing your portfolio. For instance, if you are required to submit a portfolio for a university course that demonstrates your learning over time, you may wish to structure your portfolio chronologically, while ensuring you also have a final reflection that explains the major themes of your learning.

If, however, you plan to develop a portfolio in response to audit requirements by a regulatory authority, it is important to consider that the regulators will evaluate your portfolio against the professional standards that bind your practice. In this example, those reviewing your work will know about the statutory requirements for your profession, and it is your responsibility to ensure you provide the best available evidence that demonstrates your knowledge, skills and practice. Therefore, there is little need for you to explain the regulations that inform and guide your practice; instead, you must demonstrate that you are aware of the range of regulations and give examples that illustrate your application of these in the clinical setting.

Similarly, when applying for a job the most important information to obtain is the job description and selection criteria. Without these, you may be offering knowledge and skills that do not match what the employer is seeking. A common frustration for selection or assessment panels is searching for the right information in order to appoint or allocate a pass to an application. This frustration also occurs for panels when otherwise suitable applicants who do not address the required criteria are rejected for interview or appointment. Thus, it is in your best interests to show early in the portfolio the criteria that you will be addressing – hence the value of a showcase/achievement portfolio.

Using outcomes statements, such as professional standards, learning outcomes, competency statements or standards for practice, quickly directs the portfolio reader's attention to your ability to identify and address key criteria. Once you have decided on the section headings, your main task will be to bring your evidence together and place it in the correct spots. In addition, you will, of course, need to develop a summarising statement justifying how your evidence meets the criteria. Some institutions may refer to these summarising statements as 'reflections'. A word of caution, though: this can be misleading, as the statement requires a high level of professional reflection based on a knowledge of contemporary and professional literature. While this requirement for a summarising statement may seem a little onerous, keep in mind that the structure/section headings are there to assist you, and the prerequisite skills are similar to those used in any professional documentation.

We will address how to collate your evidence and develop the narrative in later chapters of this book. For now, the focus will be on establishing the purpose of your portfolio, as well as developing an outline of a convincing argument about why your evidence of achievements meets your portfolio objectives.

What is the specific purpose of my portfolio?

The purpose of your portfolio is likely to be part of an educational assessment, position application, renewal of licence to practise, promotion application, application for exemption or credit in current studies based on recognition of prior learning (RPL), or an application to a regulatory authority for professional status. In producing the portfolio product, there will usually be some criteria to use as the structure for that version of your portfolio. Remember that the aim of a portfolio is to provide an audit trail of reasoning to support the arguments or claims of achievement made in your portfolio. Where there are set criteria, it makes sense to use these as the headings and subheadings in your portfolio. For this reason, it is imperative that you

check whether such criteria exist and that you fully understand what they mean. The selection criteria that will guide you in designing your portfolio framework are generally available via the internet, an organisation's human resources department or an educational course coordinator. In some instances, further explanation is available through online documents; for example, the various National Boards that are part of the AHPRA produce a range of useful resources in addition to the standards for registration and standards for practice. Examples of these codes, guidelines and decision-making frameworks can be found on the website of your relevant professional regulatory body.

SUMMARY POINTS

- Portfolios may be paper-based or in electronic form.
- They provide a repository space for the portfolio author to collect information and evidence and to process and develop particular skills. They also enable the production of various forms of portfolios to be made available to different audiences.
- Portfolios communicate a message to the reader, so it is important to understand and decide on the specific purpose of each version of your portfolio, including who will be reading and evaluating it.

ACTIVITY: BUILDING YOUR PORTFOLIO

If you have not done so previously, make notes now about why you are thinking of developing a portfolio and for what purpose.

- What is the reason you are putting together a portfolio? Is your portfolio for your personal use? If so, is it for you to plan your career or attend to your personal learning goals?
- Are you planning to use your portfolio as evidence to seek or maintain registration?
- Is your portfolio part of an assignment for an educational program? If so, what are the objectives or assessment criteria that will direct your portfolio construction? A common aim of assessments that require the development of a portfolio is showing that you have the skills to develop evidence of your learning. Think about the sort of picture you plan to paint of yourself as a student or practitioner.

Use a single sentence to explain the purpose of your portfolio. Then consider the following:

- What outcomes do you need to demonstrate – standards for practice statements, performance standards, role specifications, etc.?
- Who is your audience? Who will be evaluating this portfolio, and what will they need to know?

Privacy, confidentiality and disclosure

Healthcare practitioners have important legal and ethical responsibilities with regard to privacy, confidentiality and disclosure. The fundamental principles of privacy address open and transparent management of personal information, collection, use and disclosure of information, accuracy in information quality, security, and access for individuals to their own information (Office of the Australian Information Commissioner 2019). Australia has specific national privacy legislation, as well as various amendments, state and territory legislation, and industry codes and guidelines, resulting in complex regulation of privacy for both the government and private sectors (Office of the Australian Information Commissioner 2019).

For the health sector, the obligations of providers as specified in the Privacy Acts are expected to complement professional and ethical obligations regarding confidentiality contained in the various professional codes of ethics and conduct. Healthcare consumers are entitled to expect that all health practitioners will maintain a high standard of confidentiality – disclosing information to others only for the purposes of treatment (Australian Commission on Safety and Quality in Health Care 2012).

The implications of privacy laws when compiling a professional portfolio are that careful attention must be given to protecting the identities of anyone mentioned in the portfolio. Patient/client information may not be used in a portfolio unless the client has consented and the employing/placement organisation/education provider approves. Where information can be used, names of persons need to be removed or changed. In some cases, you may also need to change the details of an event or situation so that a person or persons cannot be identified. For example, if you include a case study or care plan in your portfolio, it is not only the name of the patient but also the names of the family, doctors and other health providers that need to be removed or changed. Individuals should not be named in a portfolio unless fictitiously and a statement should be made explaining that all identifying features have been removed or changed. Depending on the context of what

is being written about, there may also be circumstances in which organisations need to be de-identified. However, if someone provides you with a signed document such as a reference or performance assessment, it is appropriate for this person's name and title to be detailed in your portfolio.

Another consideration when compiling a portfolio is personal disclosure. We have suggested that you consider carefully the audience of your portfolio to ensure you send the right message to the readers. You also need to protect your own interests in the information you share. Any document you submit for professional reasons – either for assessment as part of a course or performance review, or re-licensing as a health professional – may be scrutinised by a number of people and in some cases may become the property of others. While your information should not be used for any additional purpose without your consent, it is useful to remember that there are processes such as subpoenas and freedom of information applications by which documents can be released to the public, the media or the courts. You are therefore advised to think carefully about the written disclosure of personal reflections, opinions about events or people, and personal diaries used to record work-related matters.

Organisation and presentation of portfolios

Previously, portfolios were most often associated with bulky binder folders and plastic sleeves. Certainly, the developing and evolving nature of portfolios necessitates the movement of information and, as previously discussed, the use of computers and the development of e-portfolios has changed this process considerably. We would therefore recommend to anyone starting out that you consider developing your portfolio in the format of electronic files. This will require a little extra work initially in getting or developing a template and learning how to scan the necessary documents (e.g. hand-written appraisals). The initial inconvenience will, however, become insignificant when you come to store, assemble and share your portfolio in electronic form.

Whether you compile your information electronically or in a binder folder, a neat professional product is the objective. A title page, table of contents, clear sections, and so forth, are standard requirements. The example of a portfolio structure given in Box 2.1 may be useful to consider.

The objective of Box 2.1 is to provide you with a visual sense of what might be included in a portfolio. As you can see, a portfolio has the potential to be a substantial document. However, do not be fooled into thinking that volume equates to quality: quite the contrary – a voluminous portfolio filled with certificates may communicate an inability to evaluate and discern relevance and worth. The aim is to provide concise evidence that you are competent to practise in your particular role, or the one you are aiming to work in, so the focus needs to be on the relevant competencies or standards, with the evidence and argument for how you meet them (College of Occupational Therapists of Nova Scotia 2015). As will be illustrated in the following chapters, the quality of the various portfolio entries is important in communicating an understanding of quality practice.

In moving on to consider what a portfolio might look like, it is useful to understand more about electronic portfolios (or e-portfolios) and how these might differ from paper-based approaches.

E-portfolios

We now move on to extend the introduction to e-portfolios. The focus is on examining the differences in using the electronic medium to produce and manage portfolios for learning and showcasing achievements. A key feature that will be discussed is the role of reflection in shaping portfolios regardless of the portfolio medium. It would be a mistake to assume that by using an e-portfolio, the technology will remove or reduce the need to reflect on your practice or learning. If you find

Box 2.1	Example portfolio structure

1. Table of contents
2. Portfolio explanation – details of the purpose and use of the portfolio
3. Personal details – this may be extended into personal profiles/curriculum vitae
4. Practice context, including current role descriptions and practice activities – or, if you are an undergraduate student, placement-experience record/work-experience summary
5. Standards for practice or competency statements (not listed and dependent on portfolio purpose)
6. Appendices such as:
   - professional self-assessment activity
   - professional learning plan
   - learning objectives and associated achievements
   - employment summaries
   - role descriptions
   - professional practice assessment forms
   - relevant assignments
   - medication calculation assessments
   - certificates of attainment (e.g. manual handling, cardiopulmonary resuscitation)
   - completed clinical skills assessment checklists
   - summaries of activities/tasks undertaken
   - academic transcripts
   - referee reports and testimonials
   - other relevant work-related documents.

yourself merely following a menu and uploading files without considering the connections between your achievements, your learning and your future goals, then you need to ask yourself, 'Is this really a portfolio activity?' This warning is not intended to put you off e-portfolios; rather, it is intended to highlight that there is the potential for some institutions/organisations to misuse the term 'e-portfolio' to include the uploading of files with no inherent reflective process. It is important to note that using the electronic medium to store, structure and present portfolios does provide different opportunities and challenges from paper-based approaches. In addition to including digital/electronically mediated files such as video clips, blog entries and online learning tools, e-portfolio platforms also include search facilities to manage files, plus templates to structure and present your work. Learner-centred individualised learning, lifelong learning and reflection are central to e-portfolio development (Joyes et al. 2010).

With the advent of the e-learning and associated e-portfolio industries, e-portfolios are becoming commonplace in education programs and institutional regulatory processes. Hence, it is important that you understand the benefits and pitfalls of e-portfolios to enable you to reflect critically on the value and application of this burgeoning field.

The emergence of e-learning and the associated technologies to support personalised online learning has reignited the enthusiasm for portfolio learning and in effect initiated the e-portfolio industry. Within the context of this book, the term 'e-portfolio' will be used to describe the various components of a professional portfolio undertaken electronically. More specific terms such as 'e-portfolio platform' will be used to describe the associated software programs marketed to support portfolio activities online. The term 'e-tools' will refer to the learning and other professional activities that can be used to develop and record portfolio artefacts via the online medium. The portfolio displayed online in a web page format, with embedded web links and other electronically mediated information, will be referred to as a web-folio.

Fig. 2.1 illustrates the potential components of an e-portfolio. As the figure shows, an e-portfolio software program/platform may include an array of components to support reflection and capture achievements. Online learning journals and blogs should only be used to capture reflection related to learning issues, needs and outcomes. There are many e-portfolio software programs available to support the electronic construction, storage and display of the various portfolio components. In most instances, individuals are able to access these

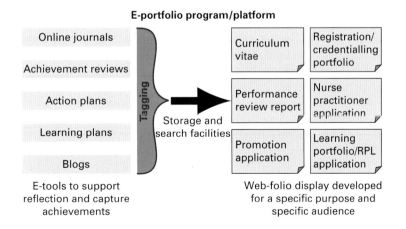

Figure 2.1 Schematic representation of e-portfolio components
(André 2010, p. 121)

programs for a fee or as part of Open Source software program arrangements. Education providers may also provide students enrolled in their programs with access to e-portfolio software. Each program has a different emphasis and may or may not include the specific components displayed in Fig. 2.1.

E-portfolio programs also provide a convenient space/repository to save your work in a space-efficient form. Depending on the program, this information can be stored locally, such as on a personal computer and data stick, or remotely via a secure server.

It is possible for an individual to put together an e-portfolio without using a specific e-portfolio program. For instance, there are numerous personal web pages used by individuals to display their learning and achievements that are quite separate from a formal e-portfolio software program. As many educational institutions have identified, however, formal platforms provide useful supports and structure for students to develop their skills and understandings associated with portfolio activities. In effect, e-portfolio platforms can become personal learning spaces, where individuals can develop their learning independently from formal educational input, store artefacts developed in educational and professional environments, and then use these to plan and design future learning opportunities.

It is not the purpose of this text to provide recommendations for e-portfolio platforms. However, by understanding the general functions of e-portfolios, you will be in a good position to decide upon a program that addresses your needs. Components depicted in Fig. 2.1 will be addressed further in the following materials.

What are e-tools?

An important facility of most e-portfolio platforms is the ability of students/users to invite others to view and comment on their e-tool products, other artefacts or web-folio pages. The convenience of doing this online, plus the security of invitation processes, is an important feature of the e-learning experience. Sharing information with others must occur with care. The ease of sharing material comes with inherent risks and responsibilities. In some instances, artefacts may be developed online in collaboration with peers, and submitted for assessment.

Some e-tools, such as wikis and blogs, include facilities to generate reports about the contributions of group members, which can be used as part of the assessment and conflict resolution processes.

A link to a wiki or blog site in your portfolio can then be a demonstration of your leadership, critical thinking and analysis, collaborative practice or any number of professional competencies. Which e-tools you might need is clearly a personal decision. Increasingly, there are some important blog and wiki sites where professionals can exchange ideas and support group learning. Professional blogs and wikis may have restricted access to allow only those invited to contribute to access the site. Setting up a blog or wiki is quite simple; the costs vary according to the size of the site and the level of access restriction. Hence, setting up a 'community of practice' for a group of clinical specialists can be readily achievable. Transferring e-portfolios to paper will mean that links to these sorts of activities will be lost. The interactive and collaborative nature of a blog or wiki site provides a level of professional authenticity that cannot be easily demonstrated in a paper-based artefact. A web link is meaningless unless accessed; therefore, if you are converting your portfolio to a paper form, you may need to include excerpts from the site as an appendix. While not totally satisfactory, this would still be a very useful artefact. It is also important to consider the perspectives of others on a closed site when you share a link. Doing so may not be appropriate.

Although not completely necessary, you can also use an e-journal to record and reflect upon your thoughts and extended readings.

RESOURCES

There are several journalling software programs available – for example, LifeJournal (www.lifejournal.com), The Journal (www.davidrm.com/thejournal) and iPhone/iPad applications.

In addition to providing the facility to write quickly and legibly, these applications/programs can include functions such as voice recording and voice recognition software, tagging and search facilities to recall materials, and prompts to encourage deeper reflection. Any note-taking system can also be used to record thoughts and reflections. These become particularly useful when associated with e-books and e-libraries, where you can search and tag information from multiple sources, embed references and structure your own reflective journal. Selective links to these facilities, or selective excerpts from these journals, can be stored within your e-portfolio repository and inserted within a specific portfolio/web-folio as a demonstration of your reflective skills applied to practice.

For those of you familiar with the use of concept maps to cluster and conceptualise information, programs such as MindManager are useful. If, however, you do not use concept maps often enough to justify the cost of purchasing a specific software program, photographing the map you have drawn on your whiteboard, or converting your hand-drawn paper versions to a PDF, can be equally useful. A PowerPoint slide or Word document offer other alternatives. Constructing a concept map can be useful in reflecting on and structuring complex tasks. The map also provides an important artefact that demonstrates your thinking in a succinct 'snapshot'.

All of the e-tools listed here have the potential to support the user in undertaking reflective activities and producing artefacts that illustrate a depth and complexity of professional practice. As previously mentioned, it is not necessary to use e-tools to achieve this; however, the benefits of the collegial exchange, ease of use and authentication aspects may well tempt you to consider including one or more of these in your repertoire in specific situations. The ease with which information can now be shared can be problematic as well as beneficial. When working on a collaborative activity, others have a stake in the outcome and may also have expectations around privacy as well. These are important considerations before sharing with third parties.

What is tagging?

One of the advantages of an e-portfolio platform is that it provides a repository for the user to save and store digital artefacts (otherwise referred to as items of evidence). Documents such as learning plans, performance review reports and presentations can be saved directly

as Word documents, PDFs or even as links to external websites. Similarly, digital recordings, and reflective blogs relevant to your learning can also be saved for later use within your e-portfolio. Over time, there can be quite an accumulation of artefacts and it can be difficult to remember the relevance of each. The facility to tag each item and then search according to these tags is therefore very useful. The beauty of a good e-portfolio facility is that each item of evidence can have multiple tags, which is quite logical as a single item of evidence can address a range of different professional criteria. The facility to store and draw upon artefacts you have collected over time is also useful in reflecting on past learning or achievement in order to better understand and map future learning and development.

As previously mentioned, the e-portfolio platform allows the user to attach multiple tags for a single artefact. For example, you could tag an artefact according to the year produced, the level of confidentiality it requires, and any number of professional competencies or role description headings. The aim is to capture whatever the artefact demonstrates, as well as to start to include issues you want to address. This will then enable the portfolio producer – or maybe, with permission, the portfolio audience – to undertake a search according to specific tags or codes.

Tagging items of evidence for your portfolio is similar to research coding. It is a form of analysis that, at one level, aims to help overcome the challenges when compiling and later drawing on large amounts of information. At another level, tagging or coding gives meaning to each of the items and explains how these items relate to each other and to the objective of producing a portfolio. Tagging your information is a useful starting point for your reflection on the relevance of a new item. For instance, imagine you have just completed your annual performance review. What tag might you attach to it as you upload it? Clearly, there are the obvious ones to do with the year and the fact that it is a performance review document. But what about the content? Is there any relationship to any professional standards, position or promotion criteria? As you can see from this example, tagging can show your thinking about how the various items of evidence relate to your professional principles and practice regulation. As a consequence, it pays to think carefully about the way you tag your evidence, as it can have a significant impact on the quality of your future portfolios. This is why some clear thinking about the purpose of your portfolio and an understanding of models (such as process and product) will help you to manage your evidence at the early (as well as later) stages of portfolio development. The activities at the end of the chapter will direct you in creating your portfolio and understanding the implications of this for an e-portfolio.

It is very useful to consider your 'tag' categories early when developing your portfolio catalogue. When doing so, it is useful to consider the likely purpose of future portfolios – for example, for accreditation, position and promotion applications, and performance review documents. Given this, the categories associated with each of these are a likely source of tag categories. Examples of this would be:

- professional competency standards
- performance review categories
- the year the artefact was produced
- common position/promotion selection criteria
- links to your professional development plan.

As previously identified, an e-portfolio platform can provide a useful repository to store items in a space-efficient form, either locally, such as on a personal computer and data stick, or remotely, via a secure server site/cloud that can be readily accessed at different locations. In some respects, this 'repository' is a computer-based filing cabinet. The tagging and search facility is a useful way of keeping track of the various items, and of accessing them quickly and conveniently when developing a new portfolio for a specific audience.

Display function – for a specific purpose and specific audience

As has already been emphasised, when producing a portfolio to display to an audience it is particularly important to consider the purpose of the portfolio. As we progress through our careers, we will need to produce different portfolios for different reasons. A promotion application is quite different from an application for recognition of prior learning, for example. An e-portfolio platform is useful in the construction of different portfolios for different purposes. Most platforms also provide a secure site to invite an audience to view your work. The following section will provide an overview of what a web-folio is and the benefits of using this approach. As has been previously identified, however, many institutions have yet to engage fully with digital and computer technology and so currently require paper-based portfolio submissions. As noted, this will reduce some of the benefits of using hyperlinks to live, reputable sites; however, with a little work you will be able to produce a credible portfolio document that draws on an array of artefacts to substantiate the claims made.

A web-folio is a portfolio displayed as a website, with a combination of headings, text explanations and embedded digital artefacts to provide evidence to support the claims being made. There are any number of websites available that readily show the components and possible appearance of a web-folio. A quick online search can help you to understand how a web-folio might look, including the possible variations. Most web pages also contain text explanations that provide the context and meaning of the content. Hyperlinks and pictures within the text provide ready access to evidence and related sites. Designing your own web-folio/website format is not overly difficult, particularly if using an e-portfolio platform that includes facilities to assist.

Most website development and e-portfolio programs provide facilities to structure your page and limit site access to invited guests. Ensuring you have appropriate privacy settings in place is very important. It is vital that information you share can only be seen by those you choose to share it with. In addition to providing valuable security and design assistance, having your artefacts stored within these sites reduces the problems of file size and audience access. It is, however, important to save your artefacts using software that is readily accessible to others. For instance, PDF and Adobe software are commonly used for this purpose.

As with any portfolio, the structure and content of a web-folio needs to support the portfolio purpose, such that the audiences are able to grasp the relevant information quickly. Headings that address the essential criteria, for example, are a useful structural approach. It is important that explanations are provided about the claims being made and the relevance of the specific artefacts used to substantiate these claims. Unlike a paper-based portfolio, there is no need for appendices; rather, the artefacts are inserted either directly (e.g. photos within the text) or as hyperlinks that then take the reader to the specific artefact. These links allow the reviewer to readily access and evaluate the artefacts as they move through your presentation.

Some institutions, universities and other educational institutions, in particular, have developed templates to assist e-portfolio users to develop their web-folios. In addition to enhancing the professionalism of the production, these templates may also assist the user to structure their portfolio and argument to suit the intended purpose. Hence, institutions are likely to develop several templates, each one addressing a different portfolio purpose. There is potential for these institutionally generated templates to include pre-populated information such as individuals' details, university grades and clinical reports. Those of you who have had to cut and paste information laboriously between performance review documents would no doubt appreciate the convenience of having some of this background information preloaded. This facility not only supports consistency in portfolio formats but also, by having the background information preloaded, enables students and employees to focus on the reflective tasks of planning and framing their argument.

The artefact repository and search function is clearly a useful facility in producing the various web-folios/portfolios. As previously mentioned, no matter the format, an argument about the learning attained or performance demonstrated needs to be made in order for a portfolio to achieve its purpose. Reviewing all the artefacts within a specific category is a useful way to contemplate the argument that might be generated. From a learning perspective, it is useful to revise artefacts that you produced early in your development, and to reflect on the learning that has since been achieved. Similarly, the argument of competence can be framed as a progressive and culminating achievement. In doing so, you are communicating the application of generic skills such as a commitment and ability to develop as a professional. Hence, reflecting on the scope, quality and progression of the artefacts you have collected is a useful exercise when considering the text that will support the various items of evidence within your portfolio.

Sometimes it is necessary to develop a paper-based or Microsoft Word document portfolio from an e-portfolio repository or web-folio, which will mean that some of the value and accessibility of the digital data is lost. In this situation, using an e-portfolio platform to develop, store and retrieve artefacts is still a valuable exercise. As previously explained, e-tools can provide useful supports in producing structured and reflective artefacts, though unfortunately audio and video artefacts provide a particular challenge if you are required to make a document-based portfolio submission. The storage and retrieval capacities of an e-portfolio platform are also a very convenient way of managing and accessing your information. All of these facilities can still be useful in developing your paper-based portfolio. The real difference is that, rather than embedding your artefacts as hyperlinks within your portfolio text, you will need to include them as appendices.

Depending on the institutional requirements, it may not be possible to submit sound and video footage; however, printed versions of blog sites, e-journal entries, documents and PowerPoint slides are all achievable. At times it may be appropriate to include hyperlink addresses, particularly if this is an external source that provides verification of your achievement, such as an online journal article or conference presentation. As previously noted, while it is disappointing that there are times when a web-folio cannot be used, it is possible to take advantage of the convenience of an e-portfolio platform and yet produce a documents-based portfolio submission.

Issues with/limitations of e-portfolios

Yes, e-portfolios have their limitations. If you were hoping that this technology was somehow going to produce a well structured reflective portfolio after a few button clicks then, alas, you will be disappointed. While e-portfolio platforms provide a convenient way to develop, store and retrieve artefacts and structure web-folios, it can be a mistake to associate this with simplifying the cognitive and reflective practices in developing and maintaining a portfolio. Ideally, as students are introduced to portfolios within their programs of study, they will be supported progressively and incrementally to develop the skills and understandings associated with portfolio learning and development.

However, while this support may assist these students, they too will be required to undertake contemplative and reflective exercises in producing their portfolio products. The real value of using a portfolio is the individualised and applied learning/profession extension that is achieved as part of the process. Unfortunately, technology has not, as yet, replaced the work needed to achieve this.

As many educational institutions have recognised in setting up e-portfolio platforms, ease of use and reliability of the technology is an absolute prerequisite. Complicated processes, non-intuitive instructions and failures in the technology, while increasingly less of an issue, are all potential risks when using an e-portfolio platform. If you are intending to use an e-portfolio platform, it is important to select one that meets your specific needs, abilities and resources. Most platforms are relatively reliable; however, problems do occur when working on underpowered computers or accessing online information via inadequate bandwidths. If you are trialling a product, it is recommended that you try uploading a range of files from the computer you intend to use. Also, be prepared to spend some time in learning the requirements of the program. Most programs come with instructional text and videos; four or five sessions of 30 minutes each should be adequate to be able to undertake most activities.

Moving between platforms can also be irritating and time-consuming. For this reason, most educational institutions provide students with e-portfolio access after graduation, sometimes at a small fee. However, it is possible in most instances to transfer files to another platform if need be. Unfortunately, this can be time-consuming and cumbersome, so you might want to consider this when deciding on a platform.

Social networking and other online environments have the potential for misuse and, as in any environment, bullying, misuse of others' work, breaches of confidentiality and other forms of professional misconduct are all potential problems. However, possibly as a consequence of a misplaced sense of anonymity, ease of access or lack of understanding, breaches of netiquette (online etiquette) are unfortunately a problem. Breaches of confidentiality and other forms of unprofessional conduct, while possible in any situation, are easily exploited and communicated to others in the online environment, and so it is important to consider your own professional conduct online and to protect yourself from the misconduct of others.

When circulating your portfolio artefacts or web-folios online, try to use PDF documents rather than Word files that can more easily be copied, used and altered. While not a complete deterrent to the knowledgeable individual who can convert PDF materials into standard text, this would be a breach of professional protocol. Also, be particularly careful about the standard of your work, do not use the work of others uncited, and ensure that the confidentiality of your clients, colleagues and institution is maintained.

It is important that your audience is also aware of their responsibilities about netiquette, providing quality feedback and not misusing other people's materials. Most institutions have policies about misuse of intellectual property; so, if you are working in a professional environment, you should have a level of protection. Unfortunately, theft of others' work does occur in all environments and the accessibility of materials in the online environment makes this a particular problem. Most institutions will insert disclaimers about this within the e-portfolio templates. The codes of conduct, through the relevant regulation Board, are also relevant in the online environment (Australian Health Practitioner Regulation Agency 2014). Issues of confidentiality, professional accountability to maintain standards of practice, and ethical requirements to protect others apply in all professional settings. In addition to understanding this for yourself, if developing your own blogs or other professional exchange environments, it would be useful to consider including a policy statement drawing others' attention to this. It is important to highlight the professional purpose of such a site and to reinforce the standard professional responsibilities of using a resource only for its intended purpose, ensuring that submissions and responses maintain the rights of all individuals, and highlighting the responsibility of others in monitoring and managing these standards. While the people with administrative responsibilities for blogs or other social networking sites have specific responsibilities to act when a breach of professional conduct occurs on their own site, we all have a professional responsibility not to sanction misconduct.

If not managed well, assembling e-portfolio artefacts and web-folios can be time-consuming and irrelevant activities. It can be tempting for those who enjoy computer-based activities to spend considerable time compiling numerous irrelevant and poorly structured artefacts in the mistaken belief that quantity equates with quality. It is important to remember that a portfolio need not include every possible item; rather, it should be a sample of your best and most relevant work. While it is important to engage with new technologies, it is equally important not to be a victim of e-gimmickry. It is disappointing to read a portfolio that is full of 'bling and ping' but short on content and process.

SUMMARY POINTS

Benefits of e-portfolios include:

- the use of diverse artefact forms including audiovisual displays and blog activities that provide more comprehensive and authentic depiction of performance outcomes, online access, storage and retrieval mechanisms.

Challenges and potential risks of e-portfolios include:

- ease of sharing can result in inappropriate or inadvertent distribution of portfolio material that can breach privacy, confidentiality, or be misappropriated by others
- the potential to be distracted by the technology such that the exercise can be time consuming.

Steps and responsibilities in portfolio development and use

Table 2.1 (overleaf) offers a series of steps to take when developing a portfolio. They would be the same whether the portfolio was electronic, web-based or presented as a hard copy. The table also suggests how responsibility for portfolio development and use might be shared between those who prescribe, require and evaluate the portfolio and those who develop it.

Two examples of different types of portfolios are presented in Tables 2.2 and 2.3. In the first example, a portfolio is developed as part of an application for a job promotion. In the second example, a portfolio is developed as part of an application to a nursing and midwifery authority for nurse practitioner status. (The principles apply to all health professionals.) It is recommended that you spend some time considering both of these because, by examining a range of portfolios, you will come to understand the specifics of your own portfolio needs.

The aim of this chapter was for you to consider the format that might best suit your portfolio purpose. The array of portfolio literature and formats available is potentially confusing.

The use of digital technologies within a professional portfolio can support learning and better illustrate the breadth and depth of professional achievements than can a paper-based portfolio alone. It is important to note, however, that an e-portfolio platform is not just about storing and retrieving digital artefacts; in many

ACTIVITY: E-PORTFOLIOS

To learn more about e-portfolios, search for the term online. If you are enrolled in a university course or program, open the university homepage and enter the word 'e-portfolios'. Most universities now offer some version of the e-portfolio for their students. Sometimes it is linked at the program or course level, while at other times resources are available through career development services. If you are not a student, search for e-portfolio information and examples through reputable search engines and follow the links. Evaluate each e-portfolio possibility for access, functionality and most importantly privacy settings.

TABLE 2.1

Steps and responsibilities in portfolio development

Stage	What is required?	Who is responsible?
Identification	Identify current practice or prior learning. This should include knowledge, skills, values and attitudes.	Portfolio developer
Comprehension and application	Describe how the knowledge, skills and values fit with the required standard. This standard may be in the form of course or learning objectives, professional standards, or a relevant role or position description.	Portfolio developer
Analysis and synthesis	Document the information necessary to communicate how the different examples of learning and practice come together into a claim, or series of claims, of achievement. These claims would be grounded in, and supported by, evidence.	Portfolio developer with assistance from guidelines or advice from the course, employment or regulatory authority staff
Evaluation	Determine the extent of learning or achievement in relation to standards or objectives. Decide whether this is a necessary or acceptable standard.	Portfolio developer (before submission), or if submitted: course, employment or regulatory authority staff (after submission)
Recognition	Recognise and register achievement such as a pass mark, employment, or registration or certification for practice.	Organisation, then portfolio developer if additional documentation or document upload is required

TABLE 2.2

Portfolio to accompany a promotion application

What is the specific purpose of this portfolio – including implications?	The objective of this portfolio is to support an application for job/position promotion. Therefore, the promotion criteria and job description are important elements to consider in the portfolio design – you need to decide which of these to use as your framework, or whether to use and perhaps combine both.
	Having read carefully the application statement or requirements and spoken to the chair of the selection committee, you may decide to use the promotion criteria as a framework, but to use bold italics whenever addressing components of the new job description. You could also make reference to the overlap between these two criteria, because this indicates insight into the position and promotion requirements.
Who will be reading it – including implications?	In a promotion application, it is likely to be the selection or promotion committee members who will read the application and portfolio. They can be assumed to be familiar with the details and requirements of the employing organisation; hence, there may be no need for explanation of the promotion criteria. Where there is representation from other departments or, in some cases, other organisations or disciplines, they may not be as familiar with the professional regulatory requirements specific to this position. In this case, it may be best to clarify your understanding of these requirements in a sentence or two.

TABLE 2.3
Portfolio in application for nurse practitioner status

What is the specific purpose of this portfolio – including implications?	The objective of this type of portfolio is to support an application for a designated role that carries a particular and high-level status – nurse practitioner. The nursing and midwifery regulatory authorities' nurse practitioner standards and any specified guidelines will need to be obvious as section headings in the portfolio. Please see Nurse Practitioner Standards for Practice (Nursing and Midwifery Board of Australia 2014). Note this document was updated in 2018. Also see Competencies for the Nurse Practitioner Scope of Practice (Nursing Council of New Zealand 2017).
Who will be reading it – including implications?	Panel members will have been nominated by the relevant regulatory authority committee appointed to review such applications. What are their fields of expertise? Do you think they are familiar with your specialty area? Might they have been nominated to the committee because of their educational and regulatory experience? Answers to all these questions will shape the information you need to provide and the format of the portfolio.

respects, it can become more of a personal learning environment.

E-portfolios do not replace all aspects of learning and skill development; however, they do provide a useful adjunct to traditional learning methods. By utilising the benefits of digital artefacts, self-evaluation, plus the storage and retrieval capacities of e-portfolios, the possibilities for students to undertake individualised learning are enhanced. The use of web-folios that demonstrate overall performance or learning provide important capstone learning opportunities, where students are able to understand the relevance of the components of a program of study. This is similar to the experience of compiling a promotion application, for example, where through the process the applicant comes to understand how the various achievements have the potential to be built into a larger picture of their competence.

 ## ACTIVITY: PORTFOLIO MODELS AND STRUCTURE

The following activities are a continuation of the learning in this chapter and have been designed to help you build your portfolio. Chapters 3 and 6 will help you to consider the content of your portfolio, including the concepts of quality of evidence.

- Look at the information you have already generated. How is this stored and organised? Are your items stored chronologically with evidence of reflection and learning directed at a specific and recent experience or event?
- Is this information ready for sharing with others, with evidence of practice standards or learning achievements evident?
- Which external audiences would require access to your portfolio, and what information from them do you need before you can prepare your portfolio?

Chapter 3

Reflection and reflective practice

Introduction

- You are aware of the requirement to be a reflective practitioner, but how does a portfolio assist you in achieving and demonstrating this?
- What reflective tools might you use to contribute to your portfolio?
- How might you reflect on your overall achievements in order to extend your learning, make a claim of competence or plan your career?

It is generally accepted that reflecting on and learning from our experience is useful in living a happy and successful life. For health practitioners, and despite limited evidence, it is also accepted that actively building integrated knowledge bases that link new knowledge to existing knowledge throughout their working lives is important in developing professional identity, and is fundamental to achieving the required standards of safety and quality of care.

The purpose of this chapter is to assist readers in understanding and applying reflection techniques in their professional development, learning, and portfolio development and use. This will be achieved through a focused overview on being a reflective practitioner. It is anticipated that this text will assist you in selecting (or possibly developing your own) reflective approaches relevant to the activity you wish to undertake.

In order to support you in achieving this, the first section of the text will provide the 'big picture' of the meaning and uses of reflection within professional practice and the relationship between reflection and learning.

Reflection within professional practice, learning and portfolios

The 'ability to self-reflect, analyse personal professional strengths and weaknesses concerning knowledge, skills and behaviours at any given moment in time, in any practice setting, is a key requirement for the caring professions' (Sezer et al. 2015, p. 188). One of the most common uses of the term 'reflection' today is as a way of thinking, a thought, idea or opinion formed from looking back and pondering (Asselin et al. 2012).

You probably have met people whose years of experience do not reflect a high level of personal or extended learning; for example, they may be good at certain tasks but lack the ability to problem-solve or understand the perspectives of others. The ability to self-reflect and analyse personal and professional strengths and weaknesses concerning knowledge, skills and behaviours is a key requirement of professional practice (Sezer et al. 2015). Reflection requires a level of contemplation or 'cognitive acts' to help broaden and deepen a person's learning. Learning results from reaching a new perspective on an event. Activities that make us think and reconsider the meaning of events are integral to the reflective process. An important component, as noted by Asselin et al. (2012, p. 911) 'of the reflective process involved the emotional responses of nurses who emerged out of and were linked to a clinical situation, … and it is the emotional component that has been missing in the previous work on reflection of nurses in practice'. Therefore reflective activities or interactions are encouraged to first recognise any emotional connection where it served to trigger a reflection. Activities should be structured in a manner that allows ideas, beliefs and knowledge to be interrogated in order to make sense of a situation and understand it more fully. These can include individual writing activities such as essays and reflective journals, or group interactions such as verbal and written exchanges with a reflective partner, journal club or community of practice. Through reflection, we learn to understand ourselves and the perspectives of others, and to extend our knowledge repertoire by engaging with and applying disciplinary knowledge.

This learning needs to be applied to practice. To do this, we need to consider all of the possible solutions and apply the most appropriate one for the specific context. Reflection on professional practice is not a personal self-indulgence; rather, it is generally regarded as essential in developing the capacity to adapt to change and thus to enhance professional practice (Sezer et al. 2015).

This process of drawing on experiences in a deliberate manner in order to enhance our understanding and consider our options for the future has a clear relationship with how we practise in the clinical environment, how we learn in practice, and how we plan and communicate our achievements. Hence, the terms 'reflective practice', 'reflective practitioner', 'reflective learning' and 'reflective portfolios' are commonly used in the professional context. Reflective practice includes examining one's own experiences, thoughts, feelings, actions and knowledge to enrich professional practice (Dubé & Ducharme 2015). Reflective practitioners, for instance, are recognised as individuals who draw on their understanding of how they interact with their environment in order to build upon their knowledge and skills, with the broader objective of enhancing the standard of client care (Jasper et al. 2013). Similarly, the term 'reflective learning' is used to describe the process of drawing on experience to contemplate the meaning, relevance and need for further learning, again with the intent to influence practice standards/approaches in the future.

The analytical aspects of reflection are also necessary when contemplating and framing an argument about competency or other achievements. In order to provide an accurate and substantive argument of achievement, it is necessary to consider or reflect on the evidence of our performance (including omissions in this evidence), contemplate the meaning of the evidence (or lack of it), and frame an argument that communicates and substantiates the conclusions arrived at through the insights gained (André & Heartfield 2007).

As previously indicated, it is the objective of this chapter to support the application of reflection in your professional development, learning and communication of performance outcomes. Portfolios, if used appropriately, are useful tools to assist both in achieving greater levels of reflection and in communicating your achievement of reflective practice and learning. An understanding of the general principles and theoretical assertions that underlie the concepts of reflective practice and reflective learning will assist you in maximising the value of your reflective activities and will be discussed next.

Reflective practice

The various approaches to reflection are based on the premise that 'we learn by doing and realising what came of what we did' (Dewey 1938 in Jasper et al.

2013, p. 43), and therefore as Jasper et al. states (2013, p. 42) 'reflective learning is the process of learning from our experiences, reconsidering and rethinking our previous knowledge and adding the new learning to our knowledge base to inform our practice'.

A fundamental aspect of reflective learning, therefore, is that we need to find ways of stepping back from situations to examine the full breadth of information, question assumptions and consider the full range of options. On a more personal level, we also need to recognise how our own feelings, actions and perceptions may have impacted upon the situation. In addition to needing to acknowledge our contribution to a given situation, reflective writers argue, we also have a responsibility to act on insights we gain through the reflective process, including the need to change our own behaviours (Caldwell & Grobbel 2013, Jasper et al. 2013).

Understanding that the purpose of reflection is to have us consider a situation from a range of perspectives is very important in understanding and valuing the reflective process. Consequently, I would encourage you to review the scenario on the next page describing a situation when reflective processes are *not* utilised.

As the exercise demonstrates, situations where reflective thinking is not used can result in limited, and possibly ineffective, solutions being proposed. In addition to wasting time and resources, situations such as this can be frustrating to work in and can contribute to an unfulfilling work environment for staff. A clinical context where health practitioners are encouraged to reflect and discover new insights will support an environment of learning and development, which contributes to greater staff satisfaction and productivity (Cioffi 2015).

What makes a reflective practitioner?

A defining feature of a reflective practitioner is the use of deliberate and considered approaches in order to examine one's own practice and question routines, with the objective of providing quality services. As Jasper et al. highlights (2013, p. 45) 'reflective practitioners are constantly moving and changing their practice as they add

> ### SUMMARY POINTS
>
> - It is often human nature to want to jump to a single solution without considering all the issues and questioning a range of social, professional and personal norms.
> - Reflection is a deliberate and structured process of drawing on past events to understand what has happened and to question otherwise accepted norms, in order to consider a range of possible actions prior to selecting the most appropriate action for the specific situation.
> - Reflection is the basis of reflective learning, reflective practice and career/professional development planning.

in the learning gained from their experiences'. Individual accountability for professional practice extends beyond the need to be able to understand and justify current actions; it includes responding to change and planning for the future. In order to do this, individuals need to reflect upon the current and future healthcare provision and needs of their client group and then have the skills to identify their learning needs, access relevant learning resources and apply the outcomes of learning to practice. There is evidence that the sense of self-determination and professional control associated with reflection supports workplace satisfaction, self-confidence and workplace integrity (Cioffi 2015, Jasper et al. 2013).

In order to respond and improve client care, reflective practitioners need to apply a combination of formal or theoretical knowledge, process skills and personal understandings (Benner et al. 2010). Formal knowledge is discipline- and specialty-specific knowledge, such as that relating to physiotherapy or to nursing and midwifery. Discipline-based knowledge is continually developing and expanding through research and professional initiatives such as the development of standards of practice. It is the responsibility of all professionals to keep themselves informed of changes in their disciplinary knowledge through engaging with relevant journals and recently published works, professional conferences and other professional development activities. As Chapter 4

ACTIVITY

Reflect upon the following scenario. Although the scenario depicts a nursing context, the process of reflection can be applied by any health practitioner. The questions listed under the headings 'Contemplation stage' and 'Solution stage' have been designed to help you consider the omissions in the reflective process and to understand the impact of those omissions.

Scenario

Belinda delivers staff development and graduate support programs at a large metropolitan hospital. At a planning meeting, a nurse manager complains that there is inadequate depth of nursing/midwifery experience to staff the night duty roster. She attributes this to a lack of undergraduate preparation and a failing of the graduate support program to prepare new graduates for this sort of work early enough. Belinda is given the brief to develop and deliver a staff development session to enable new graduates to work night duty shifts earlier in their employment.

For this exercise, we are not disputing the cause attributed to the problems, nor the solution suggested; rather, we are examining the omissions in the reflective process and the impacts this may have.

Contemplation stage

Do you think that the group gave sufficient attention to contemplating the issues that might have contributed to the lack of staff able to work night duty? Were there other possible causes/issues that needed to be considered before suggesting that new graduates needed to be the solution?

Solution stage

What are the problems in jumping to a single solution in a situation such as this? What other solutions might have been considered?

The following are some questions that might otherwise have been asked at the contemplation stage. Compare them with the ones you listed.

- What is the work environment of night duty like? Is it reasonable to expect junior staff to manage in this environment with limited support?
- What sorts of skills do staff need in order to work in this isolated setting?
- How representative is the current staff profile in addressing these needs? Is there some way of providing incentives and support for experienced staff to work night duty?

If these questions were asked, then other solutions, such as the following, might have been considered at the solution stage:

- Provide retention incentives for experienced staff to remain on staff.
- Provide incentives for senior staff to work night duty; for instance, set rosters and additional holiday roliof over school holidays.
- Provide additional supervision support for staff on night duty.

Recall one or more situations you have experienced where limited evidence has been used to justify a supposed solution. How might the outcome have been different if a more reflective approach had been used?

explains, portfolio evidence and arguments need to demonstrate a commitment to contemporary and evidence-based practice in order to be acceptable.

Process skills are necessary in order effectively to access, utilise and evaluate disciplinary knowledge. Clinical reasoning, problem-solving, teamwork, research and communication skills are all forms of process skills (Benner et al. 2010). Process skills have commonly been referred to as 'generic skills' because they are a skill set that is shared by all professionals. For instance, the discipline knowledge may differ between nurses, midwives and other health professions; however, skills such as problem-solving, communication and teamwork are necessary professional skills independent of discipline.

Personal understanding relates to how we understand ourselves and how we contribute to or influence outcomes and situations (Dubé & Ducharme 2015). For instance, professionals have a responsibility to understand and manage how they best learn, what motivates them to perform well, how they apply the regulators' code of conduct/ethics to their practice as well as how they react in a range of given situations.

As has been explained above, reflective practitioners use deliberate and considered approaches to examine their practice and question otherwise taken-for-granted routines in order to enact effective change, in both the short and the long term. It is through individuals reflecting on, and using, their formal knowledge, process skills and self-understanding that they actively develop and expand on their knowledge and skills to support improvements in client care.

Reflective learning processes will assist to unlock the learning within. It is, however, not enough to reflect but to take the next step to take action and to make some sort of change to practice as a result of the reflective learning (Jasper et al. 2013).

How does reflection relate to learning?

Learning from experience and developing reflective skills in practice is an important requirement in becoming an expert practitioner. A useful learning theory to support learning within and from experience has been developed by David Kolb, in what is referred to as 'experiential learning' (Kolb 1984). Experiential learning is an approach that enables individuals and others to recognise formal and non-formal learning within a practice context. As Pearce (2003) identifies, the values of Kolb's model of experiential learning, whereby links are made between formal learning, workplace learning and personal development, reflect the important principles that portfolios represent. It is, therefore, useful to understand the principles and practices of experiential learning in order to best utilise your portfolio. For this reason, this approach will be elaborated upon more fully here.

Experiential learning examined

The premise of experiential learning is that quality learning is achieved via using experience as a basis for reflection and application. As in the much-quoted words of the Chinese philosopher Confucius (551–479 BC), 'Tell me and I will forget, show me and I may remember, involve me and I will understand'. The need to be involved in order to understand, and the importance of this to deep and applied learning, has clearly been well understood for some time. It is through such deep and applied learning that students and practitioners understand the consequence and rationales of their actions. A useful indicator that quality learning has occurred is being able to demonstrate skills in a practice environment and to explain:

- the reasons for the actions undertaken
- the intended outcomes of the action
- the alternatives considered when deciding on the best way to proceed
- the potential repercussions that would be monitored for.

The above explanations are probably familiar to most of us as these are common questions that supervising staff are likely to ask students or novices in the clinical environment. Assessing for applied understanding is important both to stimulate this deeper learning and to ensure the provision of safe and professional practice in changing circumstances. As a consequence, experiential learning, and hence these sorts of questions, are commonly used in clinical learning environments.

Experiential learning is based on the following principles:

- For learning to be meaningful, it must result in changes to practice and behaviours.
- By seeing the value and impact of our learning, we are motivated to learn further.
- Quality learning can be achieved equally in formal and informal learning environments once an individual has developed effective learning skills.
- Individuals need to be open and ready to learn. This requires us to be able to engage in self-critique and feedback, and to be prepared to change our behaviours.
- Learning is enhanced in supportive environments that encourage honesty and respect, and value innovation and change (Jasper et al. 2013).

There are several depictions of the experiential learning model, each explaining a cycle of events that includes some form of experience, reflection and application to practice. The one shown in Fig. 3.1 (below) is commonly associated with Kolb, but he himself gives credit to Kurt Lewin for the basic design (Kolb 1984, p. 21).

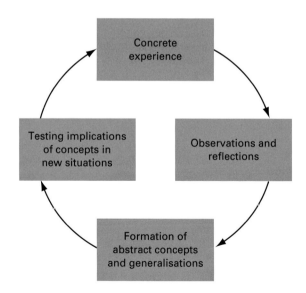

Figure 3.1 The Lewinian experiential learning model

(Kolb 1984, p. 21)

As Kolb identifies, reflection is an effective approach for recognising and integrating formal learning with informal learning through practice. In order to achieve this, the learner needs to reflect on their practice/experience in a considered manner in order to support the formation of a conceptual understanding that can be generalised beyond the specific experience. This concept then needs to be tested/attempted in practice, and this application of theory to practice then provides a further concrete experience to reflect upon (Kolb 1984). The relationship between practice application and theoretical concepts is an important one for professional learning, as conceptual frameworks enable the generalisation of knowledge beyond single specific incidents. While it may be appropriate to train semi-skilled workers to follow task lists, the very nature of a professional role requires a level of understanding to support the ability to predict and respond to change.

The following activity has been designed to help you understand how the experiential learning model might be used in practice.

SUMMARY POINTS

- Reflective practitioners are accountable for the current and future care they provide, and therefore need to examine their practice and question routines, with the objective of providing quality services.
- Clinical knowledge is a combination of theoretical knowledge, process skills and personal understandings.
- It is through practice-based experience and associated reflections that people make sense of how meaningful some learning is, based on how useful it is to them in practice.
- Reflection is initially a conscious and deliberate activity, but with practice it becomes an unconscious, automatic process embedded in expert practice.
- The experiential learning model is an approach used by novice clinicians to develop reflective skills through applying a structured framework of drawing on concrete experiences to observe and reflect, formulate abstract concepts, and then test the implications of these concepts in new situations.

ACTIVITY

Reflect on the following scenario and identify the four components in the model, namely:

1 concrete experience
2 observation and reflection
3 abstract concept and generalisation
4 testing implications of concepts in new situations.

Scenario

Deborah is a 24-year-old woman who has recently had her first baby. Belinda, the midwife caring for her, notices that Deborah is very agitated when dealing with her baby. In one instance, Belinda was called away while Deborah was bathing her baby. When Belinda returned she found the baby naked in its cot and Deborah in her bed saying she had become panicky, dizzy and unable to breathe. Later, when she had recovered, Deborah explained that she had felt like this before when presented with stressful situations. She explained that she had previously managed her anxiety by removing herself from the situation for a few minutes, and that she was usually able to 'gather herself together' and deal with the situation. Deborah explained that she could manage most emergency situations and that her behaviour was 'no big deal'. She specifically asked Belinda not to mention it to anyone, as she said she was able to manage.

That evening, Belinda reviewed the literature about anxiety disorders and panic attacks and noted that Deborah was showing many of the clinical features. As part of this reading, Belinda also noted that there is a co-morbid relationship between anxiety disorders and depression, with a considerable overlap in the clinical features. When considering a course of action, Belinda reflected on her limited role and experience in diagnosing and treating psychological disorders, but also understood that if Deborah did suffer from a form of anxiety or depression and if she was left untreated, her condition could worsen, with potentially serious implications.

Within her reading, Belinda also noted that those with anxiety disorders often felt they were being scrutinised and judged by others, and that an important part of the treatment was to enable individuals to overcome their fears in a supportive and non-judgemental environment. Therefore, she decided to proceed carefully, trying to involve Deborah in the decision-making process, thus maintaining her trust and setting the scene for a therapeutic relationship with her in the future. The next day, Belinda spent time with Deborah, gently explaining the benefits of early assessment and intervention in situations such as hers. Deborah agreed to see a clinical psychologist and they were able to make an appointment for the following day.

Reflections

Use the following headings to structure your reflections about the above scenario:

• Concrete experience
• Observation and reflection
• Abstract concept and generalisation
• Testing implications of concepts in new situations

While there is no absolute correct answer as to the components of the experiential learning model within the above scenario, the following are the authors' reflections on this scenario.

There is some overlap between the concrete experience of this scenario (Belinda observing Deborah's behaviours) and the observation and reflection (talking to Deborah after the bathing event and reflecting on this and information from the literature). Belinda's review of the literature that evening allowed her to engage in further reflection in order to move into the formation of abstract concepts and generalisations – namely, conceptualising:

- the need to act due to the potential seriousness of the situation
- the need to act in a manner that would foster patient-centred care through self-determination and trust and thus support future therapy.

Speaking to Deborah the following day was a form of testing the implications of these concepts in new situations; in particular, Belinda enacted a trusting and supportive relationship with her client in order to further her care. This, then, forms the next concrete experience and commences the cycle again.

As has been discussed in this section, reflective learning is an important part of professional learning and development, as the focus is on changing and enhancing practice. This involves reflection at levels beyond only the descriptive and including both positive and negative experiences. The experiential learning model is a useful reflective framework to guide professional learning, as a central tenet is the integration of formal learning and application to practice. By using practice to understand what we need to learn, and to understand the relevance of our learning, we are able to direct and justify our professional development needs, and hence act in a self-determining and professionally extending manner.

Tools for reflection

As has been discussed in Chapter 1, portfolios provide a useful educational tool to document workplace learning and professional development processes. Work-based learning promotes meaningful learning that incorporates the individual learning needs of practitioners to meet the demands of role development with the needs of the organisation (Jasper et al. 2013). A portfolio captures these learnings.

As a reminder, a quality portfolio is all of the following:

- a storage space (collection of artefacts)
- a workspace (collection plus reflection)
- a showcase (selection, summative reflection and presentation) (Barrett 2007).

Importantly, reflection is what 'makes' a portfolio. Without the reflective component, a portfolio is merely a 'work log'. The reflective aspect allows you to create a whole story about your achievements, drawing on work-related issues demonstrating insight and self-understanding. The real value of a portfolio lies in the reflection and learning that are generated from the activities, including the meta-cognitive act of framing an argument of achievement that draws on the various recorded activities. It is through this reflection and integration of formal and informal learning that portfolios enhance links between education, work and personal development, and make processes associated with accountability and responsibility of care more apparent and meaningful.

Reflective tools, either within the portfolio framework or independently accessed, are particularly important in introducing and structuring reflection for both novice practitioners and experienced staff.

All reflective activities/tools have some or all of the following components:

- They draw on some form of experience; this can be formal learning, workplace experience or similar.
- They use a framework to support you in describing the experience from various perspectives, critically analysing it to question your assumptions and challenge habitual thinking.

- They conceptualise/map ideas and develop a systematic plan of how and what is to be implemented.
- They implement the plan, apply ideas to practice and evaluate the impact (Taylor 2006).

So, what is the best tool/approach to use? There is an array of reflective tools used in education and practice, each with differing qualities and contexts of use. Broad approaches, such as the experiential learning model explained earlier, are particularly useful in structuring and reflecting learning activities. Other more focused approaches support more specific outcomes, such as structured personal reflections, critical incident analysis or the development of a learning plan. It is important to understand the basic intent of various approaches, and to select or develop an appropriate tool for your specific task.

As you develop your reflection skills, you will need to draw on a range of tools and approaches in order to demonstrate a breadth of skills and achievements. To select the most appropriate approach for an activity, you might like to consider the following:

- What is the purpose of this reflective activity in this specific situation?
- What resources do I have to achieve the purpose?
- How will I know if I have a quality product at the end?

There are many reasons for reflection; however, for the most part the purpose of a reflective activity will include some or all of the following:

- to support effective learning that incorporates questioning practices, considering a range of options and implementing a possible solution
- to learn from clinical situations
- to consider how best to apply formal learning outcomes to practice
- to plan your learning needs, performance review or career plan
- to engage others in evaluating or developing your practice.

A range of tools, based on each of these categories, has been included later in this chapter. For the time being, however, it is important to consider the conditions necessary to assist you to learn through reflection. These conditions include:

- *Preparation:* be prepared to engage in opportunities for reflection. Initially, this might feel contrived and awkward; however, with practice you will come to see the benefits and the process becomes easier.
- *Understanding:* you need to understand the goals and expectations of reflection – namely, to contemplate given situations in order to (1) better understand the situation and taken-for-granted assumptions, (2) consider all options, and (3) act upon the outcomes.
- *Time:* give yourself time to stop, think and reflect on situations.
- *Objectivity and honesty:* you need to develop an objective stance where you step back from your interpretations of situations and be honest about your influence and the impact of your actions. It is important to have an open, non-defensive attitude to the experience.
- *Deeper levels of meaning:* be prepared to consider the deeper meaning of moral, ethical, social and/or professional issues (Branch & Paranjape 2002) in addition to your emotional response (Monash University 2010).

Learning from a clinical/practice situation

It is important to select specific aspects of your practice to reflect upon. In particular, identify situations that are unusual or significant in some way that provide you with a learning opportunity. The significance of a situation might be that it occurs often and needs improvement (frequent and low impact), or that it is an unusual event with major ramifications (infrequent with high impact). Both positive and negative events can provide useful learning situations. Be sure to select a situation that is relevant to your learning. For instance, if you are inexperienced in managing aggressive clients in the workplace, you might choose to focus on an incident that was managed well by a more experienced staff member.

Having selected the situation, you need to select a tool or activity to help with your reflection process. It is important that this is an active process that provides a record of your reflections. While we may feel comforted that our thoughts and daydreams are well structured and deeply contemplative, in reality when you try to recall these thoughts you may well find that this has not been the case. The process of writing is a useful way to structure and justify our thinking that requires us to focus our attention, order our thoughts, and make causal and explanatory connections (Jasper et al. 2013). The permanent record of the written word also assists us to return to these thoughts for the purposes of further extension or, importantly, when constructing a portfolio to be submitted for some form of assessment, or to use as evidence of competence or an achievement.

Reflective writing

The following is a basic introduction to reflective writing approaches. There are many high-quality texts dedicated to the development of reflective writing skills that extend well beyond the information that appears here (see, for example, Bulman & Schutz 2008, Jasper et al. 2013). Most university programs also include support for students in how to develop and structure your writing, which may be useful if you require further assistance.

Writing is an interesting process as it focuses and centres our attention and thoughts. For many people, it takes time to appreciate the process of writing, as we can feel threatened by setting down our ideas and work for others to read. However, as professionals, it is important that we engage with the exercise of writing, for it is a very useful tool to help us make contact with our unexamined thoughts and create connections with new information (Jasper et al. 2013). The tangible nature of the written word is part of the benefit of writing reflectively. This allows us to revisit our written work, discuss it with others or use it as evidence in our portfolios.

As Jasper et al. (2013, p. 86) describes, reflective writing is a particular form of writing 'that is done for the purposes of learning' by exploring a subject in depth. While reflective journals are commonly associated with reflective writing, other approaches also meet this criterion, including formal essays, blog entries, or a summary written as part of your clinical performance self-assessment. The various strategies for reflective writing have been described as being on a continuum

from highly analytical, such as a critical incident analysis, through to highly creative acts, such as writing poetry (Jasper et al. 2013). It is important that you choose the appropriate approach, one that enables you to achieve the outcome you intend. For instance, a reflective journal is a useful way to understand yourself and how you interact with your professional environment, whereas a 'strengths, weaknesses, opportunities and threats (SWOT)' analysis is more focused towards developing and instigating an action plan. The following are a few focused strategies that may assist you in understanding and selecting a reflective writing approach that best suits your task. If you are intending to include any reflective writing component into your professional portfolio you must be mindful as to whom you will share it with. This is to ensure that you do not breach your professional and legal responsibilities to client confidentiality and privacy.

Reflective journal or blog entry

As previously mentioned, using a reflective journal can be a useful approach to structure our thoughts about an event or a series of events. Increasingly, individuals are using blogs for this purpose, either choosing to keep their online blog entries private or seeking feedback with a limited or extended audience of blog users. However, it is very important to carefully consider the information that you include in any reflective journal or blog to ensure that you meet the relevant health practitioner regulators' expectations as provided in their code of conduct and any relevant state or territory privacy legislation.

Whether using pen and paper or computer technologies, it is important to structure your entries to support the reflective process.

There are many ways to construct your reflective journal or online blog entries. The Gibbs reflective cycle has been selected here, as it has the benefit of dealing with both events and the feelings that the experience generates (Bulman 2008a). By understanding the feelings we associate with certain situations, we are better able to understand how our perceptions are influenced by our emotions, and through this understanding we are more likely to be more perceptive about the experiences of others. For instance, by understanding how angry we were in a particular situation we are more likely to be able to stop and reflect on the intent of others, and consider that their intent may not have been malicious. Understanding our emotions is, however, not the only focus. Gibbs's complete reflective cycle is illustrated in Fig. 3.2.

When using any reflective approach, it is important to be aware that there are levels of reflection, and that deeper levels of reflection will assist us to achieve a more resilient outcome. For instance, when using the above reflective cycle, it is important to consider the following:

- When recording your description of the event, refrain from making judgements or reaching conclusions; rather, describe the events as objectively as you can.
- Similarly, in the feelings component, force yourself to describe how you felt and focus on this before moving to the evaluation and analysis component. Also, include in here how others might have felt.
- In the evaluation section, list all the positive and negative aspects of the experience. This helps put the event into perspective, and assists those who are at risk of over- or under-reacting to a situation.
- The analysis section is where you start to make sense of the situation. Contemplate all the possible causes or impacting variables that may have contributed to the situation. Do not limit yourself to the one you think is most likely, but consider all the alternatives. Past experiences, literature or other external sources may be of use here.
- As part of the conclusion, consider the likely issues that contributed to the situation and range of actions you or others might have taken that would have changed the situation.
- From this, you can develop your action plan. What would you do differently if this situation were to happen again? And, how might you prepare yourself for this? Again, do not limit your options until you have considered all the possibilities and selected the most achievable and effective plan (Bulman 2008a).

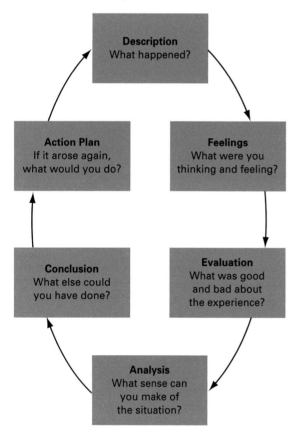

Figure 3.2 The Gibbs reflective cycle
(Gibbs et al. 1988)

Critical incident analysis

A critical incident analysis is a focused reflective activity about an incident that had meaning and learning potential. While it is common to focus on negative incidents, this need not necessarily be the case, as much can also be learnt from 'getting something right'. The analysis activity can be undertaken as a group activity, a written paper or a blog/journal entry. There are various formats or frameworks used to deconstruct and analyse an incident, including the Gibbs reflective cycle (Gibbs et al. 1988), mentioned earlier. Whatever approach is used, it is important to ask yourself questions such as:

- How might others have perceived this situation?
- Why did I interpret the situation as I did?
- Have I considered all the possible reasons for this situation occurring as it did?
- What are all of the possible actions that could have helped in this situation?
- What would I do in a similar situation in the future, and how might I prepare myself?

ACTIVITY

Select a recent significant experience and use the Gibbs reflective cycle to record and reflect upon the incident. It is recommended that you choose an experience that was very emotionally charged and significant to you. Take your time to work through the following reflective process, ensuring that you record as many details as possible. A series of questions has been included to act as prompts to help you.

Description
- What did I do?
- What did others do? What happened next?

Feelings
- How did I feel?
- How might others have felt?

Evaluation
- What was I trying to achieve?
- What was good about this experience?
- What was bad about this experience/event?

Analysis
- What are the various explanations for what happened here? How might the events have appeared from others' perspective? Having read the literature about this topic, what other explanations are there for what happened here?

Conclusions
- Having reviewed all the possibilities, what are the likely issues that contributed to this situation?
- What range of actions might you or others have taken that would have changed the situation?

Action plan
- What would I do differently if this situation were to happen again? How might I prepare myself for this?
- What outcomes will I demonstrate that indicate that I have achieved this action plan?

Having completed the above reflection, provide a brief summary of your use of the Gibbs reflective cycle.

- Did you find that the structured approach helped to draw out information that you might not have considered?
- What were the limitations of this process for you?
- How useful was this exercise in having you distance yourself from the situation and understand the perspective of others?
- Are some of the components of your action plan an extension of what you would ordinarily have learnt from this situation without the use of a reflective cycle?

Concept maps

An important aspect of reflection is the ability to conceptualise or map ideas. A concept map is a diagrammatic representation of the relationships between information and is used to structure and communicate the assimilation of clusters of information within a 'big picture' image. The basic premise of concept maps is that understanding is enhanced by relating information in a meaningful way (Schuster 2008). When developing a concept map, information is clustered into like groups and then presented pictorially to illustrate how these component groupings relate to the whole. You might be familiar with concept maps that appear as illustrations or figures within textbooks or as a slide within lectures. These maps are a useful way to illustrate the various components of a pathophysiological or other process. In most instances, concept maps are accompanied by a written or verbal explanation detailing the meaning of the illustration.

The concept map provides a useful visual summary, making it a helpful teaching tool. Fig. 3.3 illustrates a simple concept map that is referred to here as the nursing process, though it is commonly recognised as a decision-making action cycle. As those of you who are familiar with the nursing process will be aware, it gives a deceptively simplified version of what is a quite technically difficult process in practice. The simplification and pictorial depiction of the process, however, provides us with a useful learning framework to structure and inform the practice application.

In addition to providing a useful 'end' picture, the process of developing a concept map is a useful method of helping us to link new and existing information (Gaberson & Oermann 2007). Concept maps have been used to prepare care plans – for example, to conceptualise the links between the pathophysiology of a condition and the rationales of care – or to structure idea-generation exercises such as 'brainstorming' activities (Schuster 2008). Using concept maps as a method of reviewing and summarising your learning is a useful technique to prepare for exams, as, if used well, the process requires the student to engage with the content, and the map itself is a useful summary and revision tool.

The process of using a concept map to structure ideas and thinking includes the following stages:

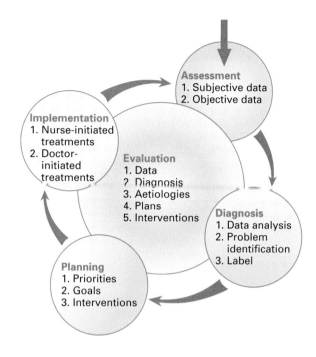

Figure 3.3   The nursing process

(Brown & Edwards 2015, p. 12)

1 purpose identification and clarification
2 idea/information generation
3 idea/information clustering
4 structuring a hierarchy of clusters.

Fig. 3.4 demonstrates the use of concept maps to design and write complex articles, such as this chapter, to elaborate on the four stages listed above. Clarifying the purpose of a concept-mapping exercise prior to commencing is important in order to maintain the focus of the exercise. If a mapping exercise does not work, it is usually because the purpose of the exercise is confused or unclear. As a consequence, a purpose statement is included within the map to clarify thinking and justify the inclusion and structuring of materials. As you will note in the concept map in Fig. 3.4, the purpose statement is written as a performance outcome or objective that explains 'what is hoped to be achieved within this article'. Having settled on a purpose statement, the salient points are recorded. During this idea-generation stage, all manner of ideas and sources are included, including reviewing the literature, colleagues'

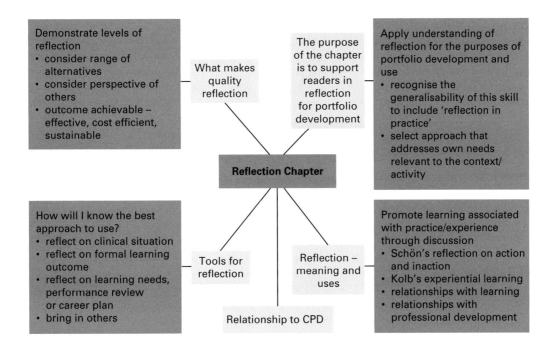

Figure 3.4 A concept map for the development of this chapter

opinions and 'brainstorming' outcomes. This stage can be quite lengthy, as it is important to consider a range of approaches and ideas prior to setting out a plan. Bring together new ideas from readings and record these on a concept map with a code that records where the idea came from. Over time, numerous isolated items of information are collected. As links start to emerge, arrows can be drawn between items, but avoid clustering information until as many new ideas as possible are recorded. When no new ideas come to light, it is time to develop the plan. At this stage, examine the relevance of various items and cluster them into groups. These clusters are groups of information about the same topic. By progressively moving between the purpose statement and the information clusters, the overall plan or map is formulated. This is the point at which to develop a hierarchical structure that explains how each of the clusters relates to each other with the overall intent of addressing the purpose statement. The diagram in Fig. 3.4, with major headings and subheadings, is in effect the plan used to write this chapter.

The figure is a simplified version of the final map that illustrates the original hierarchical structuring for this chapter. Note that the final chapter varies from this; however, the map provided an important beginning structure and allowed for more detailed writing.

While the task of writing a full book chapter is particularly complex, making a specialised software program very useful, it is possible to use a similar process for smaller activities with a whiteboard or A3 paper.

The activity overleaf draws on a concept map activity used as a staff development exercise in applying the NMBA Nursing and Midwifery Continuing Professional Development Registration Standard (Nursing and Midwifery Board of Australia 2016c). The purpose of this mapping exercise was to have the participants use the NMBA competency statements to consider the full range of possible staff learning needs within the context of their organisation. Participants were provided with the concept map structure and asked to 'brainstorm' according to each of the various categories. The reflective nature of this exercise was important in having the participants think of a range of ideas before focusing on priorities or being limited by pragmatics of what staff development opportunities already existed.

Engaging others

Engaging others in our reflections is an important strategy in broadening our perspective and gauging our own performance as compared with our peer group. Having said this, not everyone is ready to receive critique, nor

ACTIVITY

The purpose of the following exercise is for you to develop a list of possible learning needs for someone working as a registered nurse (RN) or registered midwife (RM) in your workplace (or most recent clinical placement environment, if you are a student). While not part of this activity, the intention of this exercise is that this list would assist you in formulating your learning priorities and thus contribute to your annual continuing professional development learning plan.

To complete this specific activity, for one of the practice standards, list as many relevant learning issues as you can that relate to:

- your current position description (if you are planning to apply for a promotion or position change in the near future, you might also want to include those issues that are relevant to this)
- the specific clinical environment
- changing client demographic and disease/health profiles (e.g. changes in socio-cultural or illness profile of those attending this healthcare facility)
- healthcare priorities for your institution.

For instance, if you have chosen practice standard 1, under 1.4 relating to legislation, list the legislation relevant to your RN/RM position description/role that are significant to this clinical environment. For example, a nurse manager may include aspects of industrial legislation that have less relevance to a staff member working as a level 1 RN/RM. The clinical context will also influence the relevance of some legislation; for instance, a more detailed understanding of legislation about elder abuse or food safety will be relevant to the aged care sector. Completing all seven practice standards will obviously be time-consuming, so for the time being you might want to start with just one. If you find this exercise useful, you might want to have your colleagues help you to complete the full concept map (Fig. 3.5). This list would also be relevant to any of them.

Having listed all the possible areas for one practice standard, mark an asterisk next to each item on the basis of each of the following:

- recent changes in this area (new policies, legislation or equipment)
- an area of personal weakness
- an area of increasing clinical significance (e.g. changes to your client population demographics or disease profiles)
- where a deficit in this area has resulted in a significant clinical incident in the recent past
- a significant milestone necessary for your promotion
- a set of skills needed for emergencies
- other relevant priorities.

Review those items marked with asterisks and list at least three learning priorities for the forthcoming year.

How useful was this exercise in generating a broader range of ideas that you might not have otherwise considered?

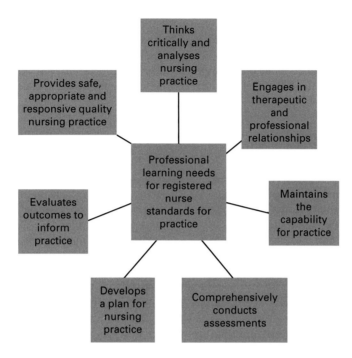

Figure 3.5 Beginning concept map for assessing learning needs against NMBA registered nurse standards for practice

(Based on NMBA 2016a)

will all our colleagues give the level and quality of critique necessary to assist us. There are times when we have some level of choice in whom we can call upon to help us with our reflection – for instance, if setting up a mentoring program, developing an online community of practice, or structuring a professional reflection group (being mindful of our regulatory and legal responsibilities regarding client privacy and confidentiality). There are, however, times when our choice of those we are able to include as part of our reflective activity is limited; for instance, generally we have little say in the appointment of our clinical supervisor or who will manage our performance appraisal process. Whatever the situation, the skills of giving and receiving feedback are very significant in making the most of these opportunities.

Why engage with others?

Having others critique and contribute to our work has the potential to expand and advance the outcome significantly. A well-structured group/relationship can assist in motivation, efficiency and the overall quality of the product of the group endeavour. Groups working together have been shown to produce more significant outcomes than if the same activity were undertaken by individuals. In other words, there are significant potential benefits in sharing your reflections and working with others to assist in your development. Groups can, however, also be ineffective, or worse, destructive to individuals. Hence, it is important to instigate strategies to support the development of positive group dynamics when setting up your peer appraisal activity, online blog or mentoring program.

How to engage with others

It is important when setting up a peer support or appraisal process that the right individuals are involved and that the 'rules of engagement' are clear and well understood. The 'right individuals' are those able and willing to critique your work and help you to develop strategies to develop professionally. You will need to make your own judgement about individuals who best meet these criteria. In some instances, your line manager or peers may have these requisite skills, while in other situations you might be better off having someone from outside your institution provide a 'fresh perspective' to your reflections. Whatever the situation, it is important to choose carefully and be clear about what you hope to achieve from the relationship.

As previously mentioned, setting the 'rules of engagement' early is also important. The following points are the sorts of details that should be discussed with your mentor at your first meeting:

- purpose and duration of the arrangement, including time commitments required
- sorts of activities to be undertaken – for example, case study reviews, debriefing exercises, etc.
- preparation commitments for each meeting; for example, will you be setting an agenda, providing a written reflection to discuss, etc.?
- confidentiality of information exchanged
- commitment to honest and productive processes, including being open to change
- a clarification of boundaries; for example, mentoring roles should not interfere with other professional relationships.

It is important to discuss the specifics of each of these rules to support a shared understanding of what they mean in practice.

An important part of engaging with others in a professional and effective manner is our commitment to providing and receiving quality feedback. Quality feedback is appropriately timed, descriptive and specific, constructive and tailored to the individual. 'Appropriately timed' can, of course, mean different things to different people; however, for the most part it means as soon as practical following the incident or episode, while taking into account the need for discretion. Descriptive, specific and constructive feedback provides the individual with a balance of sufficient details to make a more general

point, while also including direction and suggestions for change. It is important to balance positive and negative feedback, not only to make the person feel good but also to reinforce what has worked well so that this might be further replicated and developed.

The provision of feedback is not unidirectional; rather, it is an exchange of information. If we are prepared to give feedback, we should also be prepared to receive it; and vice versa: we should be prepared to give feedback if we receive it. Therefore, in any positive professional relationship, we need to invite others to provide us with feedback about our performance. In doing so, we need to accept others' comments in an attentive and non-defensive manner, encourage them to elaborate and provide details, take the information on board and make changes where appropriate, and, finally, give recognition to those who have assisted us in our development.

Conclusion

This chapter has been designed to assist in the use of reflective techniques within the professional context. It is through reflective contemplation that we are able to learn from and about practice, and thus further develop our professions. Portfolios are useful tools in both supporting and communicating professional reflection, and therefore are widely used within educational and professional recognition processes. As this chapter has discussed, there are numerous tools that can be used to support and record our professional reflections. It is important to select or develop an approach that meets the needs of a specific situation. Over the course of our careers, we will utilise numerous reflective tools and approaches as we develop our practice, plan our careers and contribute to the development of new knowledge. In addition to structuring these activities, these tools also act as artefacts or evidence that can be used when making a claim of competence or further reflecting on our achievements. As the following chapter will elaborate, we need to be cognisant of the quality and generalisability of this evidence, and ensure that our claims and proposals are accurate, robust and well supported.

Chapter 4

Evidence: What do I have and what do I need?

Introduction

- You need to start collecting items of evidence for your portfolio, but where do you start?
- How do you decide what to collect, and how do you judge the quality of the items of evidence?

Chapters 1–3 of this book addressed the 'big picture' to help you understand the overall purpose of a portfolio as a whole. Chapters 4–5 will show you how to put together the various parts of the portfolio so that its aim – to produce an account that demonstrates and evaluates progress towards learning and/or professional competence – is achieved. This chapter will introduce the concept of evidence, explore the nature of the quality of evidence, and describe how to use it to support the claims that are made within a portfolio.

A portfolio needs different types of evidence to support the claims it makes. Information about your plans, efforts, progress and achievements over time need to be brought together into a coherent structure and argument. It is this combination of evidence and a written position or argument of achievement against specified standards, objectives or criteria that allows a portfolio to achieve its determined purpose. To recap,

portfolios may be developed to record ongoing learning, professional development and achievements. They may also be created to present particular competencies, capabilities and outcomes for assessment. In the United Kingdom and New Zealand, and in some of the Health Practitioner Boards of the Australian Health Practitioner Regulation Agency, portfolios are an expected part of the registration audit process. The Boards randomly audit members of the various registers to ensure the person meets the required standards for their licence to practise. As discussed in Chapter 1, portfolios cannot prove that a person has a certain level of clinical competency. However, there is a well-established track record in nursing specifically of portfolios having a valuable role in demonstrating learning progress and outcomes, whether as a student before entry to practice or as a practising nurse (Green et al. 2014). In a well-designed portfolio, this development is evident in the reflective thinking and writing skills, as well as in other examples of evidence.

These skills, the choices made about the most suitable evidence to include, and the way in which the portfolio is structured communicate what the person understands about their professional role and responsibilities.

The following discussion explores a range of issues that are useful in building a portfolio. It is important to be clear about the aim of the portfolio. The quality of the accumulated items of evidence will, at least in part, dictate the quality of the overall portfolio. In this way, evidence acts as the 'building blocks' that provide substance to an argument of learning, achievement and/ or professional competence.

Where do I start?

Most likely, you already have some evidence from which to develop your portfolio. You may have records and experiences from your professional studies, clinical or work-based practice, and employment. Each of the courses you complete in your entry-to-practice education will have specific learning objectives that you will have demonstrated via assessment items. If you are employed as a health practitioner, your experiences will be a rich source of evidence, such as documents that describe the healthcare organisation or setting and your role. You should also have some (preferably written) feedback about your induction and performance in this role. This feedback might include a performance management or clinical assessment report or a professional reference. You will also have evidence of professional development you have undertaken. The records are part of producing an account of professional knowledge, skills and performance.

The following discussion explores the different types of evidence, how to decide what is quality evidence, and how to collect and produce the evidence to address different standards, criteria, objectives or competencies. It is important to remember that the portfolio's structure and content all need to link to its purpose. Whether a portfolio is for assessment of learning outcomes in further or higher education studies, or for performance review at work, it is always an account of what the individual has experienced and learnt, supported by evidence. The depth and breadth of this evidence is dependent on the purpose of the portfolio. A portfolio will provide

a place for you to reflect on practice and develop how you write about or record this. The results of this work will form part of your evidence. All of the evidence in a portfolio needs to enable your portfolio audience (such as an educator, lecturer, employer or manager) to have confidence that learning has occurred, and that the capability for practice (knowledge and skills) is in place and is continuously being developed. A tip is to focus on the aim and type of evidence, as well as the amount.

A reassuring reminder at this point is that, no matter what the portfolio's purpose, it is always a 'work in progress' that develops and improves over time. While versions of your professional portfolio may be extracted or produced for presentation or assessment purposes, a portfolio alone cannot prove or disprove anything. It contains the ideas and evidence to support claims made against externally assessed requirements.

To get you started on thinking about evidence, Fig. 4.1 (opposite) provides examples for practising nurses and midwives of some of the types of evidence that may be included in a portfolio (Norman 2008). While this figure is now a little dated it still provides a comprehensive range of possibilities of what might constitute evidence. It is important to remember that confidentiality requirements and organisational policy may prohibit the use and sharing of some items of evidence such as minutes of meetings or case studies in specific situations.

What is evidence, and what is its purpose in a professional portfolio?

Evidence takes many different forms, but its purpose in a professional portfolio is quite simply to provide a foundation for the claim of achievement. As we can see from Fig. 4.1, evidence is usually in the form of an object, written document, recording or a product of some sort. In the figure, the word 'Explanation' has been added to 'Evidence' in the central circle. This is because the components of the outer circles are objects that only become evidence when they have been considered and discussed in a reflective, interpretive commentary that

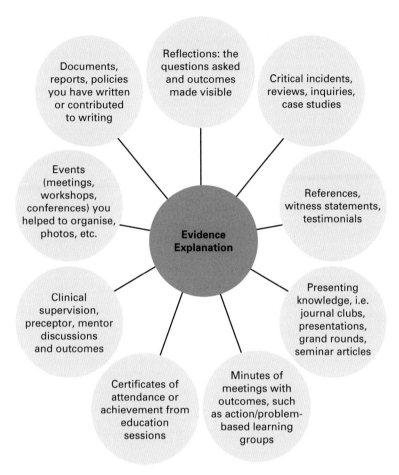

Figure 4.1 Types of evidence

(Modified from Norman 2008, p. 49)

provides justification for their inclusion in the portfolio and explains how they individually and collectively link to the overall portfolio argument of professional achievement.

In the same way that, in a legal trial, lawyers argue for the significance of particular pieces of evidence, so a portfolio needs to argue purposefully why various items can be brought together to create a particular position. For this reason, careful consideration needs to be given to the reasons for including each item of evidence in a portfolio.

Evidence-based practice may be used to argue a case for the relevance of some evidence provided in a portfolio. There are powerful empirical reasons to base healthcare decisions on research evidence, with health professionals committed to integrating the latest research evidence into their day-to-day practice in order to deliver the best possible outcomes. A range of standards and guidelines direct and influence health professionals' practice to ensure it is consumer-centred, information-driven and organised for safety (Australian Commission on Safety and Quality in Health Care 2012). Evidence-based practice for health practitioners requires them to give proper consideration to what is the best available evidence, including research findings and current practice guidelines, as well as thinking about how this evidence fits with the needs and values of the client and the available expertise (Hoffman et al. 2013). The Nursing and Midwifery Board of Australia's Standards of Practice for the Registered Nurse (2016a) foreground the ethical and relational nature of nursing and the significance of translating evidence into practice for quality outcomes. Evidence-based practice is defined in these standards as accessing and making judgements about translating the best available evidence – which includes the most current, valid and available research findings – into practice.

Although healthcare research may not provide all the information necessary to direct the full scope of actions that are undertaken by any health practitioner in providing safe and appropriate healthcare for their clients, it is fundamentally important that health practitioners know of the existing evidence for the recommended best practice related to their actions, and be able to provide sound reasons for how their actions relate to this evidence.

In addition to research evidence, information to support an explanation of evidence in a portfolio may come from other sources. These sources include other published information and people, such as professional colleagues, co-workers, clients and/or employers, managers or other authorities. Additional information can also come from personal observations, reflections and experiences.

An effective portfolio will demonstrate person- and context-specific circumstances, as well as an understanding of the impact of the relevant broader healthcare and professional contexts, such as social, political and cultural dimensions. For all health practitioners, this includes providing links that show how their practice relates to the relevant health and professional practice standards and guidelines.

The selection and use of quality portfolio evidence shows your awareness and understanding of the required capabilities for the context and level of your practice. It demonstrates that you are aware of the different characteristics of your learning or practice environments that shape your outcomes and achievements. Such evidence as workshop or course completions needs to be supplemented with a description of how you apply this knowledge in your practice. Description of the workplace context is also important. The clinical settings or other contexts in which you practise will significantly influence how you both use your existing knowledge and skills and develop new knowledge and skills. For example, although the principles may be the same, knowledge and skills in breastfeeding support will be enacted and described differently in the context of home-support programs, birthing suite or midwifery management roles. Similarly, pain management abilities will be described very differently in the contexts of emergency, community, recovery, rehabilitation, residential aged care or surgical care. Mental health intervention may be very different when the nearest specialist or inpatient facility is thousands of kilometres away, or where the patient and the mental health practitioner are both members of a small community.

Different forms of evidence serve different purposes with some serving multiple purposes: for example, a certificate in chronic disease management might be used to support more than one claim; for example, certificates for training or course completion can be evidence of achievement of learning and be supplemented by descriptions of how these competencies are used and developed in practice in a specific area. A certificate of attendance at a conference, workshop or an educational session is not in itself evidence of being competent. Levels of competency, particularly for skills, can really only be demonstrated effectively through achievement of assessment or practice outcomes as assessed by a third party. A description of your reflection on acquiring and applying new skills is a further important piece of evidence. Review Chapter 3 on reflective practice for insight into how describing, structuring and interpreting experiences or critically analysing specific incidents can improve thinking and writing skills, as well as provide lessons for future practice.

The discussion so far has outlined how the quality of items of evidence is important to the overall aim of the portfolio in demonstrating not only reflection on practice but also an informed view on what best practice is, and how your practice or learning and achievements measure up.

What is quality evidence?

Your work in bringing together the best evidence within a portfolio demonstrates a number of things. It shows your knowledge and experience in some of the necessary skills and practices for your professional role. The selection of artefacts, the framework you use to structure these examples under specific standards or criteria, and the associated rationales, explanations or learning goals can show developing understanding and abilities. Generating the evidence to communicate your practice-related abilities includes finding a way to bring together the messy contradictions that can exist in everyday practice with the relevant professional standards. The very nature of professional practice, and the associated notion of individual professional autonomy of practice, are premised on the idea that a practitioner will perform at an appropriate level in a range of circumstances, some of which have yet to be encountered (O'Connell et al. 2014). A review of competency-based frameworks found that all health professions in Australia

used some form of competency expectation to define practice and registration requirements (Brownie et al. 2011). For registered nurses, competency expectations have been renamed as standards for practice by the Nursing and Midwifery Board of Australia (2016a), and the Paramedicine Board has professional capabilities for registered paramedics. In stating what it is that the relevant health professional does in their practice, these standards indicate the level and combinations of skills, knowledge and attributes that are required. Each registered practitioner has a responsibility to interpret these standards within the dynamic contexts of their own practice scope.

Quality evidence is accurate, tangible and from a range of primary and secondary sources available at that time and over a period of time, and is able to be authenticated when necessary. Hence, when deciding if an individual item is of good quality, you need to consider the following:

- What do I want to demonstrate in this portfolio – standards, competencies or experiences?
- What is the best tangible evidence I can use to demonstrate this actual performance?
- Is this current evidence – that is, does it demonstrate my *current* practice – and is it consistent with measures of quality contemporary practice?
- Is this evidence transferable? Does it show what I have learnt and what I may do differently in the future?

The following information will assist in addressing these questions.

Tangible in nature

The definition of the word 'evidence' is associated with the need for real or tangible information. Tangible evidence is information in a form that another person can view independently in order to judge its quality and relevance. It requires being able to show that the evidence is accurate and reliably based on facts or genuine achievements, experiences or circumstances. Academic transcripts and records of attendance or contribution to continuing professional development sessions are often viewed as reliable examples of such evidence. Other examples may include meeting notes or reports showing participation in quality improvement, audit, research, human ethics, policy or practice development committees or review processes. Electronic or web-based resources might include PowerPoint, video, podcast, or online postings or presentations with records of the event, date and audience where these were presented.

While any English-language dictionary may define evidence simply as establishing the facts or reasons to believe something, evidence has different meanings in healthcare. Health professionals use many different types of information and knowledge in their practice. They also use evidence that is gained from research. Evidence-based healthcare is an attitude of inquiry that answers specific questions as the basis for providing the best care in the most resource-useful manner (Hoffman et al. 2013). It is for this reason that a professional portfolio for a health professional need not only include evidence as support for claims made about learning, competence or performance, but as suggested earlier also link to the research evidence that underpins quality healthcare practice. Healthcare practitioners may also undertake research as part of research studies, in their own practice or with colleagues, and sometimes even with clients in their care. It is important to recognise that evidence-based practice is not seeking the views of colleagues or adhering to organisational guidelines or policies where they are outdated, or where the health practitioner does not know what evidence they include or when they were last updated (Cashin et al. 2017).

Health practitioner practice becomes suitable for use in a portfolio when activities and behaviours produce planned outcomes. Direct patient and/or non-direct patient care can be observed and should be evaluated against documented standards. The considerable development in setting, using and communicating clinical outcome measures across healthcare might in some instances provide a means to map practice, though these measures may not always be easy to capture in a portfolio other than by reflective statements or peer review. The form of evidence needs to be considered carefully. For example, a team or workshop presentation may not be written up in the same way as a conference paper would be in peer-reviewed conference proceedings or a publication, but this is not to say that the examples described are not valuable evidence. Evidence that is

externally validated, such as proceedings or publications, provides verified and detailed accounts, as well as accepted endorsement of the quality of the activities described. Similarly, written notes about, or verbal recordings of, a clinical activity make the evidence item available and able to be externally assessed by others. While other tangible evidence of clinical activities includes documented health assessments, care plans, referral letters and case presentations, it may not always be possible to include such evidence in a portfolio. These items relate to individual clients and cannot be used for purposes other than service provision without their consent. Organisational policies also regulate the use of these aspects of evidence. It is very important to be aware of and adhere to the privacy laws, as well as related policies and guidelines about the use of personal information and social media. The policies and guidelines are produced and mandated by the relevant government departments, such as the Office of the Australian Information Commissioner (2019) and professional and regulatory authorities. In New Zealand, there are a number of authorities responsible under the *Health Practitioners Competence Assurance Act 2003* for the registration and oversight of practitioners in specified health professions (New Zealand Government 2019).

A behaviour becomes tangible in practice and is suitable for use in a portfolio where it produces a planned outcome that can be shown in some way. As examples, wound care, pain management and suturing are visible skills that can be observed and evaluated against expected standards. Similarly, improvements in a client's parenting skills or self-management of a chronic condition are measurable outcomes that, at least in part, demonstrate effective practice. Unfortunately, these outcomes can be difficult to capture in a portfolio. Photographs may assist in some instances and are particularly useful in recording visibly observable changes over time. For instance, with client consent it might be appropriate to photograph wound healing with de-identified digital records made of the success and appropriateness of a prescribed therapy and quality practice. Single items of evidence generally, however, have little meaning when submitted out of context. Depending on the requirements of your portfolio, this example of evidence would need to be supplemented by the inclusion of the context in the form of a more detailed case analysis or clinical report. With client consent and that of the healthcare organisation, a contextually based detailed case analysis, for example, has the potential to transform a range of relatively intangible evidence into documented form, thus allowing others indirectly to observe and evaluate. Where relevant to your area of practice, audit results can provide a useful form of tangible evidence, particularly when analysed against your role description. Audit results can also demonstrate change or development when associated with an implementation in which you have been involved.

As previously stated, issues of privacy, consent and intent are very important, and there are many obligations for employed and regulated health practitioners in this regard. Legal, organisational and professional standards and codes of conduct include consent, confidentiality and disclosure, and are designed to protect the interests of persons in hospitals and other healthcare settings. It is reasonable to assume that people in public places may be aware that they may be observed without their consent; however, health practitioners may inadvertently breach professional standards or organisational policies if they obtain and use photographs or other materials without appropriate consent. It is necessary to review the relevant directives, policies and guidelines, and to get advice from suitably well-informed colleagues, supervisors, managers or your relevant health practitioner regulatory authority if you are wanting to use such forms of evidence in your portfolio.

Primary and secondary evidence

The term 'primary evidence' is used in this book to refer to portfolio items or artefacts that are produced and developed by the practitioner for the portfolio, such as reflection on learning-outcome-related achievements and client-care activities (Jasper et al. 2013). 'Secondary evidence' already exists and is introduced into the portfolio to support claims being made such as testimonials from a supervisor or colleague or a copy of an article written for publication (Jasper et al. 2013). In a portfolio you will need a combination of both primary and secondary evidence to substantiate your claim of professional competence.

One way to communicate that your portfolio is a genuine representation of your performance is to include

evidence that is a reflective account and is substantiated by others – that is, secondary evidence. Secondary evidence may be a report of observations of practice with signed assessors' reports of the actual levels achieved, reaccreditation or test results, or a letter of support from a senior colleague substantiating the quality of the services you provide. Similarly, a client may provide a letter of support, or you may use an evaluation form to collate feedback about your performance. Some organisations encourage the use of peer evaluation/review processes; at senior levels, this may include a wider range of resources such as 360-degree feedback assessments producing useful forms of secondary evidence substantiating your claim of continuing competence.

The quality of the secondary evidence within a portfolio is judged both on what is said and on who is saying it. A quality reference needs to be provided by someone who has reason to be familiar with the quality of your work and who has expertise in the area they are commenting upon. Letters from clients are useful to substantiate claims of caring, compassion and, in some situations, currency of knowledge. These need to be mixed with letters of support from a senior colleague, however, to substantiate claims of clinical excellence and technical skill. It is important to align the evidence with the correct performance indicator.

Primary evidence, namely documents and artefacts that are products of your daily practice, need to be judged based on professional standards. As will be detailed in later chapters, when compiling a portfolio it is important to justify the way in which items of evidence demonstrate achievement of specific standards and/or competencies as they relate to best practice. Explaining the relationship between an item of evidence and these standards of practice is a vital part of the justification process. It is important, therefore, when collecting primary evidence that consideration is made as to how this might best demonstrate and meet the standards of a profession. For example, do not be tempted to include a case study that had a positive outcome if the evidence and write-up of the situation does not address the necessary course or assessment objective, standard or competency statement. It is important to evaluate the item of evidence for the skills and abilities that you can demonstrate about yourself, including your ability to problem-solve and respond to change.

A range of sources

As has been mentioned, evidence used within a portfolio must include a range of items that demonstrate aspects of professional performance. A portfolio for an experienced practitioner may include such items as an employment record linked to position descriptions, letters of support from clients and staff, journal articles or presentations, documents or client instruction sheets developed by the practitioner, and so on. Each item of evidence in the final portfolio is selected to demonstrate aspects of performance. For example, authorship of a client information handout can demonstrate a range of skills and understandings, such as the ability to write in a clear, concise and appropriate manner, taking into account the literacy skills of the client group; the inclusion of contemporary information; and the desire for client empowerment through the communication of resources and information. However, the development of a client information handout does not demonstrate a range of assessment or clinical skills, and thus there remains a need for diverse sources of information to show evidence of the range of requisite skills to meet the specific professional role.

For most health professionals, case studies, that have client and organisational consent, are an important means of demonstrating an application of clinical skills. A single case study may provide a range of portfolio items, such as the client assessment report, care plan, case analysis and more. A student or new practitioner may produce an acceptable portfolio using a single case study with other evidence items, such as undergraduate assignments, academic transcripts and clinical assessment reports. An experienced practitioner may have a routine of documenting significant or relevant critical incidents or case studies, with client consent, every three to six months, providing them with a rich resource of multiple and varied evidence to use.

If you are a student, remember to keep notes throughout your clinical or experiential placements of the various things you did and learnt each day. Remember also to record not only new things you do but also the areas where you do things with a higher level of competency – such as providing the same care without prompts or remembering to evaluate the effect of your nursing or midwifery intervention – and document them

accordingly. Such records will be invaluable when writing your portfolio. It is also important to assemble your portfolio as soon as possible after clinical or experiential placements, as the longer you wait, the more difficult it becomes to be accurate.

It is also worth thinking beyond your individual performance even though the portfolio is most likely to be used to demonstrate individual achievement. As discussed in Chapter 1, competence is most commonly considered from the individual perspective. However, evidence will exist for most health practitioners and midwives about inter-professional and team competence. These are the outcomes of a professional group to which you belong and actively contribute. With healthcare becoming increasingly complex, we understand that care is now rarely provided in absolute isolation from others. The geographically isolated rural or remote health practitioner usually has some access to technology to enable consultation with and referral to other health professionals. Recognition of patients as the experts of their own health experience also necessitates their central role in decisions about their care.

Education of health professionals about how to work together effectively has been demonstrated in a systematic review to improve some of the ways health professionals take care of patients (Reeves et al. 2013). A related idea of 'collective competence' has been studied in a number of settings, from aircraft crews to hospital staff and as part of workplace culture and organisation and relationships. Collective competence is understood to be when individuals create shared models of best practice. An example might be where health professionals on a ward or healthcare unit provide competent individual patient care while also knowing collectively what needs to be done for other patients in the ward or unit. This ability would be very familiar to experienced health practitioners and midwives who work effectively in teams and communicate at regular intervals, as well as covering each other in taking responsibility for patients to ensure that they are safe and quality care is provided while staff take breaks or manage unforeseen events. In this way, collective consciousness is more than a combination of individual competencies, with interaction a key feature. Identifying evidence that demonstrates collective competence that can be shared can be problematic. When the evidence belongs to a range of individuals all must agree to its use unless it is an artifact in the public domain.

Suitability and relevancy

Portfolio items of evidence will be assessed by the reader for their suitability and relevance to the claims of meeting standards of practice or learning objectives. Anxiety about not meeting the required outcomes or standards is a common emotional response to learning or assessment experiences. Most people feel anxious or vulnerable when making information about their work available to others for judgement. However, it is important to note that it is through taking this type of risk that changes in learning and practice occur.

The evaluation of whether an item meets contemporary standards of practice differs according to the nature of the activity. For instance, to have a paper accepted by a peer-reviewed journal or conference is in itself an affirmation that the paper meets a specific standard. With other activities, however, the assessment must be apparent through the demonstrated use of external measures. Many academic items of assessment require that students read widely and demonstrate the integration of a range of external ideas and research findings through academic referencing. Similarly, it is useful to reference the use of professional practice standards when preparing a portfolio item. If preparing a case study, for example, it is recommended that you include references to hospital protocols or the professional literature where

appropriate, thus demonstrating familiarity with, and use of, the literature. By aligning your work with practice standards, you are able to demonstrate your currency as a practitioner, and therefore the suitability and relevance of your evidence.

A primary item of evidence and indicators of quality need to be linked through reflective commentary (as discussed in Chapter 3 on reflective practice and how this can contribute to portfolios). It would not be unusual to include secondary evidence, such as a supporting letter verifying that the item being discussed is your own work and represents your usual standard.

Regarding the earlier discussion of privacy and confidentiality, it is important to reinforce that while a range of techniques and sources may be used to generate the best possible portfolio evidence, all information gathering and reporting needs to be conducted in an ethical manner. The collection of portfolio evidence must not compromise an individual's welfare or rights. This point cannot be reinforced enough. Written consent is required where a portfolio includes information about, words or images of others.

Evidence for portfolios

In Chapter 2, we described different approaches to take in structuring a portfolio. Each of the different ways shares some evidence, such as employment records and academic transcripts; however, the purpose of the

What is quality evidence?

- Tangible in nature – evidence that is genuine, may be factual and can be evaluated
- Primary and secondary – evidence that already exists, and new evidence that needs to be generated for this specific purpose
- Diverse range of sources
- Evidence that is suitable and relevant

Each item of evidence needs to be tangible in that it provides evidence of some aspect of your practice. There needs to be a range of items – some from primary sources that provide direct evidence of practice, and some from secondary sources that help substantiate the authenticity of your claims. Each item needs to demonstrate quality practice and thus, where possible, be aligned to evidence-based practice indicators.

portfolio will determine the required evidence. Table 4.1 describes examples of some of the types of evidence.

As demonstrated in the table, the type of evidence becomes more complex depending on the purpose and audience for the portfolio. For example, care must be taken in aligning items of evidence against any specific criteria, such as the regulating bodies' professional competency or practice standards. An understanding of what each of the statements means is clearly very important.

ACTIVITY

Search the web page of the relevant National Board at the Australian Health Practitioner Regulation Agency for guides to using the standards for practice for your profession. Can you list other codes, standards or guidelines that relate to your practice? Examples of these may be specialist or quality standards such as those produced by specialty practice organisations and the Australian Commission for Safety and Quality in Health Care.

Alternatively, resources to assist in understanding criteria may be available through searching the relevant literature. It is recommended that you make yourself familiar with the criteria or standards, carefully checking that you have not misinterpreted or narrowly interpreted any of the statements.

TABLE 4.1
Portfolio evidence examples

Evidence	Examples
A diverse range of documents related to your professional or educational activities and competence. These tend to be records conveniently provided by employers or educational institutions rather than deliberately developed by the nurse/midwife for the purpose of a portfolio.	Employment record Academic transcripts, awards and certificates Log of continuing educational activities (compulsory and elective) Registration record
Documents developed to demonstrate actions and competence in relation to specific outcomes or objectives. While some documents are conveniently available as a consequence of work and educational activities, others are purposefully developed to provide evidence of an identified learning outcome.	Learning log Educational activities and assignments Justification statement
Documents developed to describe previous actions and competence against predetermined competency criteria – similar to that of a process-oriented portfolio. Often these documents are *purposefully* sought or constructed to address a specific standard.	Clinical assessment record Records of other competency review processes
Documents describing previous actions against predetermined criteria as part of a broader analysis of professional competence. These documents are purposefully acquired to address a specific component or competency.	Case study (consent of others required) Publication (e.g. journal article) Presentation (e.g. conference or seminar)

Selecting evidence for a portfolio

Ask yourself what existing standards of practice, knowledge, skills and attributes (competencies) or learning outcomes you can demonstrate. If you list a series of competencies or learning outcomes, the next question is: What do I have that will allow me to demonstrate these? For each piece of evidence you think of, ask yourself the following questions:

- Is it primary or secondary evidence?
- What is the intended purpose of including this evidence?
- What standards, competency, learning outcomes, assessment criteria or experiences does it relate to and demonstrate?
- Can it be used to support or illustrate more than one criterion or achievement?
- Which reflective, analytical or interpretive point in the standard does the evidence support?
- Where in the portfolio should it be placed? (Modified from Jasper et al. 2013, p. 153)

To help you identify your existing documents and understand how they help build a portfolio, it is important to consider your portfolio's purpose, outcomes and audience. The next activity is designed to assist you to identify the items of evidence you hold and how this evidence might be described.

In most instances, a single item of evidence has the potential to address a range of activities and skills, so portfolio structure is important. Chapter 2 discussed portfolio models and structures, and the next chapter will address putting a portfolio together; however, a reminder of portfolio structure is useful at this point. Box 4.1 may assist you in visualising the components of your portfolio. Visualising the format will help you to understand the need to evaluate portfolio items for relevancy to the specific standards that make up the framework you are using to structure your portfolio. It is not unusual to accumulate a range of portfolio evidence items that address a single competency statement or component of performance and yet have insufficient items for other areas. For most health practitioners and midwives, unless they have been presenting to their peers or undertaking further studies, the experience of compiling evidence is not common. Therefore, where

Box 4.1	Example of portfolio structure

1. Personal details
2. Summarising statement
3. Standard 1
3.1. Statement of justification
3.2. Evidence summary
4. Standard 2
4.1. Statement of justification
4.2. Evidence summary
5. Onwards – continuing through each of the standards that you are using to frame your portfolio
6. Evidence items or appendices
6.1. Curriculum vitae
6.2. Academic transcript
6.3. Position description

portfolios are introduced as a requirement of professional development or regulation, it is important that this is done in association with supportive staff development and changes to performance management processes. In doing so, it is important that professional development activities are designed to provide tangible evidence that can be contributed to portfolios.

You have a range of evidence … what next?

This chapter was designed to help you identify what constitutes quality evidence. This is assessed by having a range of items of evidence, with each item being substantial and related to some aspect of your practice. Items need to be partly from primary sources that provide direct evidence of practice, and some from secondary sources that help substantiate the authenticity of your claims. Each item needs to demonstrate quality practice, and thus, where possible, be aligned to evidence-based practice indicators. As will be explored in Chapter 5, collecting a range of quality evidence items, though a vital part of compiling a quality portfolio, is only the beginning. Your next step will be to put together your evidence and match it against each of the performance

ACTIVITY

Do you have a résumé or curriculum vitae? If not, now is a good time to draft one or to review your most recent job or promotion application. Can you identify what physical evidence you could provide to show that you have achieved each item on your résumé? For example, you would have a letter of offer of appointment to show that you attained a certain position, or an academic transcript documenting completion of courses and programs. Next, list all the potential portfolio documents you have relating to your professional practice and/or learning as a student. Now consider the following:

1 What sorts of items of evidence do you have?
   a What form does the evidence take (e.g. is it something you have written, such as a case study-based assessment item, or health information brochure, or a reflective or commentary piece)?
   b What sort of evidence is it (e.g. is it 'convenient' evidence such as that provided by an employer or educational institution about compiling a portfolio, or do you have some items that would act as 'purposeful' evidence to demonstrate a process, standard or product)?
   c Think about the quality of the evidence. Using the information provided earlier in this chapter, assess your evidence in relation to the following questions:
     i How tangible is the evidence?
     ii Is it primary or secondary in nature?
     iii What are the links that show this is evidence-based practice?
     iv Does all your evidence come from one source? Are there other sources?
     v How suitable and relevant is each document?

2 How does all this evidence come together in addressing the aim of your portfolio?
   a What are the strengths and weaknesses?
   b Are there any gaps?

At this point, you may find it useful to share your information with a fellow student, work colleague, clinical supervisor or mentor to get their views on the strengths, weaknesses and potential gaps in your evidence.

3 Find and interpret the criteria that are required or might be used to assess this portfolio. It may be professional standards such as those required by a nursing and midwifery regulatory authority, assessment criteria such as those required by an educational provider, or even a position description produced by a potential new employer. Consider the match between the portfolio evidence that you currently have and the type of portfolio you are required to develop or that will best meet your needs. Where are the overlaps and gaps? Is the spread of evidence even across the criteria? Have ethical expectations, including confidentiality, been maintained?

indicators/competency statements. This will highlight any gaps in evidence you have and may require that you generate or put together additional evidence. The concept of quality evidence is central to this process, for it is only through the compilation of quality evidence that you will be able to achieve a quality portfolio.

The following activity has been designed to help you reflect on items of evidence and consider how the quality

of these might be assessed and enhanced. Further, this will assist you to understand, and hence explain, the relationship between individual items of evidence and the claim of competence being made.

This activity could be used for each item of evidence. Fig. 4.2 illustrates how this activity would relate to the multiple examples of evidence required for a portfolio. This would be a considerable amount of work and all

ACTIVITY

Select a significant item of evidence. Now use the diagram below as indicated:

- In box A, attribute this evidence to a standard or area of competency or learning.
- In box B, describe the item of evidence according to the practice activity of learning experience it demonstrates.
- In box C, list the factual information that informed your actions for the relevant item of evidence.
- In box D, provide a list of all the relevant best-practice evidence and/or professional guidelines related to this topic area/practice.

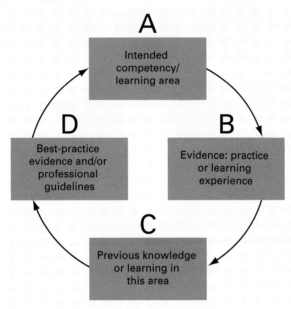

Having completed each of the boxes, reflect on the quality and relevance of the item of evidence. The following questions will assist with this.

- Is there alignment between the evidence and the standard or area of competency or learning?
- Does the evidence reflect sound knowledge and best-practice principles?
- Is this a suitable item of evidence, or could I improve upon this (e.g. would a commentary be useful in demonstrating further learning and practice development)?

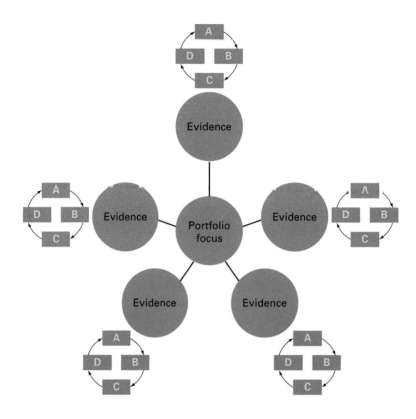

Figure 4.2 Reflecting on the quality of your evidence

of it may not always be necessary, but it is a useful exercise in identifying the foundations of current and best practice.

Conclusion

This chapter has examined the nature and purpose of quality evidence, plus how to recognise it, produce it and enhance it. Understanding how evidence informs and supports a portfolio is essential in producing a quality product, be it a claim of achievement or providing direction for learning and professional growth. Similarly, recognising the quality of individual items of evidence is necessary both in selecting those that are relevant and enhancing existing items. Having achieved this, you are now in a position to commence assembling your portfolio, where these items of evidence will be used to substantiate your claims of achievement and inform further learning.

Chapter 5

Compiling your portfolio

Introduction

- You understand the aims of a portfolio in developing reflective thinking, communicating learning and achievement in studies for entry to a health profession, and in recording practice and continuing professional development.
- You also understand the need for and features of quality evidence. You now need to consider the evidence you already have and start developing your portfolio.

This chapter will guide you in creating a portfolio, with activities to assist you included throughout the chapter. If you have not already started, we suggest that you write your insights or key points in a Word file or notebook. As you read through the chapter you can use your notes as a foundation for building sections of your portfolio. It may help if you visualise your portfolio as a book. A book has a cover, with a foreword and a table of contents (book chapters) and some may have a conclusion. If you look at the concept of a portfolio as your own 'book' it will allow you to more easily see how the smaller portfolio sections fit in the bigger picture of your larger professional portfolio.

Regardless of which of these smaller portfolio sections becomes the driver for your larger professional portfolio, we recommend designing your table of contents for the professional portfolio as an early priority to provide

scaffolding and balance, firstly for your ongoing professional development and secondly for the integrity of the overall structure of your larger professional portfolio. Also adding information regarding each of the intended portfolio sections will help to clarify the professional and personal images that you are aiming to communicate to the reader via your professional portfolio.

The production of a quality portfolio is undertaken progressively, over time, as you consider a series of interrelating steps for each of the sections of your portfolio. These steps are as follows:

1 Identify the purpose of the section of the portfolio you are about to create.
2 Select an appropriate portfolio structure for the section. In some cases, this may involve accessing a prescribed framework or template, such as that

from an employer. In others it may be a template you develop for your specific purposes such as to record your experience during a conference or study program.

3 Consider any information or evidence you have collected so far.

4 Identify gaps in your evidence and generate new evidence to address these gaps.

5 Review and organise the content of this smaller portfolio section to ensure the materials correspond to your overall larger portfolio.

Your knowledge and experience will influence how you build your portfolio sections. Consider how you will frame each portfolio section. If you commence this process and find that your approach does not work in achieving your portfolio objectives then restructure so that the overall aim for your portfolio section is achieved. Determining what will work best for documenting your professional development in each section you create often requires careful consideration.

Deciding on and designing a portfolio framework

How the sections of a portfolio are incorporated into the overall portfolio design is an important consideration. A portfolio's strength lies in organisational clarity, cross-referencing, quality evidence and quality analysis (Emden et al. 2003). In order to achieve this, it is imperative to develop a plan early in the development process (Cooper & Emden 2001). Therefore, having gained some understanding of portfolios, it will be useful for you to develop a schema of what your portfolio will look like and give you an indication of the sort of information you will need to compile and develop. As previously indicated, some professional organisations have provided ready-made portfolio formats, either in text form or via an e-portfolio interface. It is worth going to your professional organisation's website to see if they provide a portfolio format for your profession to use. To assist midwives in the compulsory competency review process for re-certification, the New Zealand College of Midwives produces and makes available for purchase structured portfolio frameworks.

The purpose of your portfolio will inform what will be the most appropriate framework to use. If your portfolio is for an application for your first job as a health practitioner, then it will be important to refer to the relevant national practice standards and match evidence of your personal and professional attributes to these. If the portfolio is for performance review by your employer, then you will need to pay close attention to the requirements of your job description.

Suggested framework for portfolio

Personal details

This first portfolio section is the same as would be included in a curriculum vitae (CV) or résumé. It may be omitted in an educational or learning portfolio. It requires a summary of your personal details, such as:

- name
- contact details – phone, email, postal address
- professional registration details
- qualifications and education
- summary of employment
- current position description
- professional memberships
- names, titles and contact details of referees.

You are likely also to choose to address broader skills, attributes, experiences or activities, such as those required by an educational or employing institution. These must be relevant to the purpose of a portfolio and should not overly duplicate material included elsewhere. A number of professional regulation authorities provide examples in various documents about competency and continuing professional development activities. It is important to check if your regulation authority has specific requirements for a portfolio structure, the type of evidence of competence to practise as well as the application of learning to practice.

A more generic example of additional items would include:

- personal career goals
- scope of practice statement

- a summary of recent continuing professional development plans and activities (including points accrued, if relevant)
- publications and/or presentations and research activities
- relevant volunteer work, or related skills and qualifications such as a first-aid certificate etc.
- police check, immunisation and health records.

Statement of learning

Summary statement of arguments or claims

The objective of an introductory statement is to give the reader a sense of the overall purpose, claims and plan of the portfolio, thus preparing them to understand the intention of the portfolio before focusing on specific details. The main purpose of this statement is to address:

- the purpose of the portfolio
- how the purpose is to be achieved
- if appropriate, the relationship between the portfolio, your current and expected scope of practice, career, and educational and learning goals.

An example of how you might start your summary statement for a portfolio framed around the Australian competency/practice standards for your relevant health profession would be as follows:

This portfolio has been designed to provide documentary evidence of my competence/practice as a registered ……….. as part of my regulatory requirements with the …………….. Board of Australia (…..) and through my scope of practice as a ……………… in the area of …………… In order to achieve this, the competency/practice domains have been used as the main framework, with examples of evidence used to demonstrate both my current performance and developing skills in the area of ………………

The above summary statement becomes a declaration of your competence to practise within the specified role and practice environment.

Alternatively, a summary statement for a course-related portfolio might read as follows:

This portfolio has been designed to provide documentary evidence of my learning as part of the course objectives and assessment requirements for the course/assessment.

The course objectives/assessment requirements have been used as a portfolio framework with examples of evidence included to demonstrate (development and outcomes).

While you are likely to need to change your summary statement as your portfolio progresses, it is useful to develop a draft statement early because this will help you to clarify the overall purpose of the exercise and start you on the way. Like the table of contents, the summary statement will provide a useful reference point for you to refer back to as you build the portfolio and select, alter and even omit materials in the final version. For example, if you find yourself struggling with sections or aspects of the portfolio, refer back to this first statement and ask yourself:

- What are my knowledge skills or abilities for which I need evidence?
- How is this material relevant to the overall aim of the portfolio?
- Which competency or aspect of learning does it address?
- Do I want to include examples about thinking, learning, operation, or practice skills or strategies?
- What makes this a quality example?

The answers to these questions will help you to clarify which materials to include and what to keep on file for future reference.

The next section goes on to discuss how to set out the evidence in the portfolio and especially in the case of a student, where they may have to demonstrate that a specific competency, practice standard or learning objective has been met.

Statement of justification for why arguments of claims can be accepted

A statement of justification is an explanation of how competence or learning has been demonstrated by detailing how the item of evidence is a demonstration of a competency statement/practice standard (see Table 5.1 for an example of a justification statement). In addition to explaining the link between the item of evidence and the competency statement or learning objective, the statement of justification details how these items are a demonstration of contemporary practice or effective learning, and hence show a level of quality achievement.

TABLE 5.1
Example: Evidence summary table with justification.

Standard or competency domain	Transcribe the relevant standard/competency domain statement here, e.g. Registered Nurses standard of practice 6.1: provides comprehensive safe, quality practice to achieve agreed goals and outcomes that are responsive to the nursing needs of people	
Statement of justification	Specify how you will be relating your evidence to your health profession's competency or practice standards, e.g. include an explanation of the concept map undertaken as it relates to competency 6.1	
Evidence statement	Title of evidence: e.g. Concept map: care of an elderly man with type 2 diabetes	Appendix number, e.g. 1

(This table may be most suitable for students who often have to deconstruct and show they understand every aspect of a competency/standard)

Evidence summary table

An evidence summary table provides a tabulated display of which items are included as evidence to support your argument of competence, where these items can be located and, if appropriate, which specific component of the competency, domain or learning objective the evidence addresses. Table 5.1 provides an example of an evidence summary table. In the first instance, use this as a working document to list the items you think appropriate, with a brief description of why they have been included. As you progress with your portfolio, this reasoning can help develop your statement of justification further.

The statement and evidence summary table with justification should be repeated for each of the required competencies/practice standards or learning objectives if required.

Appendices

The purpose of appendices is to provide supplements referred to in the main text, thus supporting the veracity of the claims being made. The benefit of certain reference items being included as appendices is that they are maintained in full, rather than being presented as excerpts within the main text. The appendices are a combination of the items of evidence you have compiled for the purpose of the portfolio that are sufficiently integral

to the portfolio purpose to warrant being included. In the case of e-portfolios, the appendices are unlikely to be at the end of the web-folio; rather, they will be embedded as links throughout. As discussed in Chapter 2, these linked items can be in a range of digital forms, including links to external sources such as best practice guidelines, national/international standards or conference proceedings (if available).

One group of portfolio appendices will need to be the items of evidence that you have compiled. With a few exceptions, the size and complexity of the items of evidence you will be compiling make it inappropriate to embed these as whole items within the portfolio because the flow or argument within the portfolio would be disrupted. An alternative to this is to embed smaller components of evidence, although this then diminishes the integrity of the evidence itself. For example, a complex item of evidence such as a case study is much more informative when available as a complete entity than when it is provided as small portions and extracts included in the broader argument. Further, these items are likely to demonstrate a range of skills and be applicable to a range of competency/standard subcategories. Thus, a case study can be referred to under several competency statements, practice standards or learning objectives, while the quality associated with the whole can be maintained by its inclusion as an appendix. Remember that it is important for the relevance of an appendix item to be clearly articulated when it is referred to.

Examples of items of evidence that may be included are as follows:

- learning objectives and associated achievements such as academic transcripts or completed case studies (see Chapter 1, page 5, regarding patient confidentiality), concept maps, and other educational assignments or presentations.
- an employment summary
- continuing professional development attendance details documented in accordance with the requirements specified in the relevant regulatory authority standards
- competency assessments, test results/certificates of attainment for completion of training or updates, such as cardiopulmonary resuscitation, medication management, emergency procedures, supervision and quality management, etc.
- performance review, professional practice or clinical supervision documentation
- presentations, publications and/or photographic records
- research proposals/applications or quality initiatives in policy development
- referee reports and testimonials.

The second group of portfolio appendices refers to supporting institutional documents that help to frame your practice. These documents might include:

- professional competency standards
- codes of ethics/conduct
- organisational policies
- role descriptions.

A cautionary note here: institutional/organisational documents should only be included if they are highly relevant and freely available to the public (see Chapter 1, page 5, regarding confidentiality).

The headings that have been suggested in this section have been incorporated into Table 5.2 (overleaf) to provide an understanding of how a product-oriented portfolio might look. You will be looking further at actually constructing your portfolio soon.

RESOURCES

Both the Australian and New Zealand health practitioner regulatory authorities recognise ongoing learning as part of their re-certification/renewal processes. It is important for you to access online the relevant standards, information and guidelines or suggested templates provided on websites by the relevant professional and regulatory authorities.

Collecting information or evidence

It is now time to compile the pre-existing evidence for your portfolio. Your most recent educational and practice-based experiences are likely to influence the type of evidence that you have readily at your disposal. When compiling your evidence, it is recommended that, if applicable, you use the competency domains or practice standards that are specific to your role.

As discussed in Chapter 3, a range of types of evidence is needed to substantiate the complex claim of competence. In particular, you will need a variety of evidence that addresses the breadth of your practice, including items from both primary and secondary sources. To recap, primary evidence refers to artefacts or texts that pre-exist as a consequence of what you have done in work, study or in practice as part of your professional activities. Examples of primary evidence include assignments. Secondary evidence refers to information that is provided by someone such as a supervisor or colleague, and may be used to substantiate claims made within the portfolio. You will need to make a judgement about how recent an item needs to be for currency; this depends on the nature of the item and your practice.

Table 5.2 (on page 66) will help you to think about the structure of your portfolio. As you will note, the items of evidence have been categorised against generic competency statements or practice standards that are

TABLE 5.2

Suggested portfolio framework or template

Personal details	Decide what should be included in the summary of your personal details, such as (delete and add as relevant): • name • contact details – phone, email, postal address • registration details • qualifications/education • employment summary • current position description • professional membership • referees' names and contact details • personal career goals • scope of practice statement • learning plan plus summary of recent continuing professional development plans and activities (and points accrued, if relevant) • publications and/or presentations • research activities • relevant volunteer work and related skills and qualifications, such as a driver's licence, first-aid certificate, etc. • police check, immunisation and health records	
Summary statement	Summarise the purpose of the portfolio and give a brief overview of how you plan to achieve this purpose:	
Standard or competency domain 1	Transcribe the relevant standard/competency domain statement here:	
Statement of justification		
Evidence statement	Title of evidence	Appendix number
Standard or competency domain 2	Transcribe the relevant standard/competency domain statement here:	
Statement of justification		
Evidence statement	Title of evidence	Appendix number
Standard or competency domain 3	Transcribe the relevant standard/competency domain statement here:	
Statement of justification		
Evidence statement	Title of evidence	Appendix number
Standard or competency domain 4	Transcribe the relevant standard/competency domain statement here:	
Statement of justification		
Evidence statement	Title of evidence	Appendix number
Appendices		

suggested to have relevance to most health professionals. We suggest you may want to create a document similar to Table 5.2 to commence the construction of your portfolio.

From the list in Table 5.2, and items you may have added yourself, select those items that are of sufficient quality and relevance to be included in your portfolio. As explained in Chapter 3, quality evidence needs to be current and represent contemporary standards of practice.

Next, you should title your pre-existing evidence and include the titles in the relevant evidence summary tables, adding notes on how each item of evidence meets the standard or competency. It is also useful at this point to list each of the items within the appendices; you may or may not wish to use numbers for the appendices at this stage as the order or appearance may change. The process of labelling and transposing information within your portfolio is simplified, as discussed in Chapter 2, if you are using an e-portfolio.

Identifying omissions and generating new evidence

Now that you have entered your items of evidence within the evidence summary tables, you will be able to identify which categories are well supported with quality evidence and where omissions exist. You will now have a basis on which to consider what evidence you will need to generate to support your wider claim of competence or that you have met your learning objectives.

How do you know how much evidence is enough? There is no single answer to this question because it depends on a range of variables, the purpose of the portfolio and your personal circumstances. The amount of evidence might be relatively small if, for instance, as a student you are required to submit a prescribed list of portfolio items as a course assessment, with the aim of the assessment being to demonstrate your applied understanding of that aspect of portfolio compilation and justification. In this case, the restricted number of evidence items requested would be sufficient. However, if you are compiling a portfolio to substantiate your learning outcomes or argument or claim of competence to perform within a specific role, something much more

substantial is required. The full scope of the relevant standards or criteria would need to be addressed within your portfolio.

The remainder of this chapter has been written for those planning to compile a comprehensive portfolio to support a claim of professional competence. Nevertheless, it will still have relevance to those developing a learning portfolio and, therefore, even if you do not wish to undertake this exercise in its entirety, we recommend that you review the process since the principles involved will inform your understanding of portfolio construction.

At this stage, it is important to re-familiarise yourself with the requirements of the organisation to which you will be submitting your portfolio. This may mean closely reviewing your key regulatory documents such as competency/practice statements, decision-making frameworks, portfolio assessment processes and/or schemas and employer requirements. It is during this process that you need to consider what these organisations value and, hence, what you need to communicate clearly through your portfolio. If, for example, your regulatory organisation provides a checklist of requirements, then it is obviously important that you follow this in detail. In most cases, however, this will be a broad guide only, with no prescriptive list detailing the type and scope of all evidence requirements for your portfolio. This is perhaps because both the nature of practice and individual professionals vary so much, and as quickly as such a guideline might be developed it would be superseded by changes in practice.

As discussed in Chapter 1, the ability to assess and articulate our own competence and scope of practice is central to self-regulation and current notions of professionalism. Health practitioners need to possess the level of competence for both day to-day practice and for the future, to remain part of the flexible and responsive health workforce. Given this, competency or practice standards, and similar regulatory guidelines, generally provide relatively broad descriptions of practice requirements, thus allowing the range of variations that sit within a health professional's practice.

So, how should you proceed? Revisit the activity at the end of Chapter 1 and review your list of competencies and/or practice standards in light of your expected scope of professional practice. Next, review your job documentation or position description. Highlight those sections you consider to be essential aspects to your role and indicative of your scope of practice. In other words, what are the important skills you use every day? What are the skills that you may use less regularly but are nevertheless essential to your role (e.g. in emergency situations associated with your role)? What are some background skills that reflect your understanding of your risk management, regulatory and professional frameworks? While a complete portfolio needs to include evidence that addresses all standards, the specifics need to reflect your own particular situation and knowledge.

Moving on with building your portfolio, we suggest you review the contents of Table 5.3 and reflect on the areas not well represented by the evidence you already have. Once you have compiled a list of the additional evidence you will need to complete your portfolio – where to next?

First, you may find that you do already have an item that will cover the area identified but had not previously seen the connection or relationship. It may be a useful exercise to see in how many places in your portfolio a particular piece of evidence can be used.

Second, consider whether you need to increase the range of evidence in your portfolio. It is also important that you select a form of evidence that best demonstrates the knowledge, skills and attitudes associated with the competency you are seeking to highlight or support. For example, a table listing the regulation that frames your practice and how this might be applied in practice is a useful way of demonstrating your associated knowledge, but not necessarily your attitudes as applied in the practice setting. An accompanying letter from your supervisor detailing your diligence in following through with your legal obligations, however, will provide the supportive evidence required. This may mean that you will need to enlist the assistance of others in compiling your portfolio evidence.

Third, you may have identified that some aspects of your practice or learning are incomplete and that you need to undertake additional training or extend aspects of your current role before you can generate the evidence required.

A fourth idea might be to share your 'work in progress' with a friend or colleague who is also a health practitioner in order to brainstorm new ideas. Alternatively, you may approach a supervisor, mentor or lecturer to get more structured feedback on strengths, limitations and gaps to assist you in moving forward to completion. You might review the nature and types of evidence to see if stronger evidence can be obtained through different forms, such as statements written by others, publications or references to your contribution elsewhere, such as in organisational, unit or committee reports.

Other questions you might use to evaluate your portfolio include:

- Are the central claims and justification statements clear and consistent throughout the document?
- Does the portfolio have both breadth and depth of evidence?
- Is there balance in the focus, sources and types of evidence and information?
- Is the portfolio discussion and evidence focused on persons (individuals and groups), actions, knowledge, skills, attitudes and values?
- What is the balance in the portfolio between creative, descriptive, factual and detailed information?
- Are there unexamined assumptions or values that need to be challenged, better explained or removed?
- What style of language has been used? Is there any jargon or vague terminology? Is it objective or subjective?
- Are terms used consistently? For example, have you described providing care to patients, clients or healthcare consumers? Which term best communicates your intentions? Have you used any specific terms or language prescribed by the regulatory authority or employing organisation?
- Are all sections useful in building the arguments and adding support, or is there padding in some sections where nothing new is being added?
- Are any statements distracting from your main purpose of the portfolio?
- Do a reality check. Does this portfolio show the best of what you have done in either your practice or learning?
- Does the portfolio hold together as a supported account of your achievements?

TABLE 5.3

Details of portfolio evidence

General categories relevant to practice standards	Examples of evidence to support claims. Which of these types of evidence do you already have or what needs to be done to get them?
Practice: in accordance with relevant: • legislation • ethics • standards/codes of conduct and practice • scope of practice/ decision-making frameworks	• Explanatory statement/table clarifying your understanding of the links between your role description, scope of practice, reporting management framework, and other legislative and policy responsibilities • Case study – needs to refer to relevant legislation, regulatory guidelines and/or institutional policies • Supportive letter that demonstrates your applied understanding and preparedness to act in an ethical, culturally competent and professionally responsible manner • Letter from insurance company or employer website address detailing current insurance cover* • Copy of annual practising certificate • Educational qualifications or professional membership for practice according to profession legislation/code of practice • Attendance at relevant workshops, conferences, seminars • Other
Communication: demonstrates relevant skills: • verbal and written • teamwork and interdisciplinary collaboration • referral mechanisms	• Professional artefacts that demonstrate written skills • Case scenarios demonstrating verbal communication skills and professional networking • Position description detailing reporting and referral mechanisms • References/testimonials provided by clients or professional colleagues detailing your communication skills • Attendance at professional development activities related to developing and using communication skills • Details of professional presentations given • Other:

Assessment and planning:
 • for individual clients and/or groups in a range of situations relevant to the context of employment or practice (e.g. emergency, multicultural perspective)
	• Position descriptions detailing client assessment responsibilities
	 • Client case studies (with evidence of patient consent) detailing assessment and plan of care, including:
	   – direct client assessment (interview and physical examination)
	   – the use of supplementary information sources in assessing the client's needs
	   – plan of care that represents both the client's needs and contemporary practice
	 • Completed assessment documentation demonstrating understanding and application of a theoretical framework/structured approach
	 • References/testimonials provided by clients or professional colleagues that include comments about your assessment and planning skills
	 • Attendance at, and participation in, relevant professional development activities
	 • Other:

Continued

TABLE 5.3

Details of portfolio evidence—cont'd

General categories relevant to practice standards	Examples of evidence to support claims. Which of these types of evidence do you already have or what needs to be done to get them?
Delivery of care: • planning and implementation of care • supervising and managing others • collaborating with an interdisciplinary healthcare team	• Position description and scope of practice statement detailing client management responsibilities • De-identified exemplars detailing plan of client care you have implemented for a range of clients/client groups • Performance review documentation detailing the quality of care you have provided while employed • Client and/or peer testimonials detailing the quality of care • An incident analysis that details your skills and performance in the delegation of care • Descriptions of health education activities undertaken • Other:
Evaluation of practice: • client outcomes and appropriate modification of care • institutional processes	• De-identified audit report (if permitted) or process related to an aspect of your practice • Supervisor's report or a performance review process commenting on your self-evaluation and client evaluation skills • Reflective analysis demonstrating a high level of self-reflection and professional critique • Exemplar detailing activities contributing to review and development of institutional policies/guidelines • Other:

Contribution to the profession:
• participation and contribution to research activities
• implementation of evidence-based practice
• professional development of self and others
	• Membership of and contribution to:
	  – professional organisations
	  – workplace committees
	  – community groups
	• Research articles or other publications
	• Details of presentations delivered
	• Literature review
	• Documents detailing educational support provided to others
	• Performance review documentation that includes comments on your skills and activities in this area
	• List of professional development activities undertaken
	• Other:

TABLE 5.3

Details of portfolio evidence—cont'd

General categories relevant to practice standards	Examples of evidence to support claims. Which of these types of evidence do you already have or what needs to be done to get them?
Personal development	The previous sections have addressed what you do in your professional practice. The focus of this section would be on demonstrating how you practise, how you develop your practice, and how you learn from experience. It would include reflective analysis of your own behaviour in the following ways: • explorations of particular patient encounters • objective reviews of your role in critical incidents or working groups such as journal clubs • analysis of how you developed your learning plan • reflections on annual performance appraisal.

Insurance cover is a regulatory requirement for some health professionals, including nurses and midwives.

- Does it hold together literally in terms of style, presentation and binding?
- Or, if you have developed an online portfolio, are the pages well constructed with active links?

There are not necessarily any right or wrong answers to these questions. The best answers will come through careful reading of your portfolio and consideration of how well it incorporates any required criteria or standards in meeting the portfolio purpose.

Conclusion

This chapter has examined how to identify, create, collect and organise evidence in a professional portfolio. Considerable detail has been provided on how to structure your portfolio, including generating your argument, producing summary and justification statements, and embedding the evidence to achieve the strongest support for your claims for learning. If you have followed the suggested steps carefully, it is likely that your last task will be simple. The final product needs to be reviewed to ensure that the arguments of achievement or statements of claim are supported and justified by the organisation and evidence within the portfolio. Chapter 6 will provide more detail and guidelines about assessing and evaluating portfolios.

Chapter **6**

Portfolio evaluation and assessment

Introduction

- You are a health professional or student developing your portfolio and want to understand better the perspective of the assessor who might be evaluating your product.
- You are a lecturer considering introducing portfolios as a student assessment.
- You are a member of an appointment or promotion committee seeking guidelines on how to assess the value of individual portfolios.

The focus of this chapter is how to design and conduct professional portfolio assessments. Portfolios are commonly used in education, professional practice and regulation as a way of sharing and evaluating the ongoing development of standards of practice and to promote the achievement of high levels of complex performance and outcomes. Associated with this, portfolios are used to promote and evaluate a health practitioner's commitment to ideals such as: ongoing professional growth and development; the application of contemporary and developing standards of practice; and professional leadership. Given this, portfolios are often the assessment of choice for applications for promotion, role extensions or continuing professional development. The benefits of portfolio assessment – namely, having the applicant draw on their practice to demonstrate current and developing professional competence and standards – is clearly very appropriate in these circumstances.

However, it is also a complex exercise, with the potential for poorly implemented evaluation and assessment to inhibit or delay the achievement of positive professional outcomes. It is the objective of this chapter to provide some ideas and advice to institute a positive and effective assessment approach when it comes to the complex issue of professional portfolios.

As this chapter details, portfolios are assessed for different reasons, and the reason will influence the appropriateness of assessment approaches. For instance, if the purpose of the assessment is to share learning between a learner or practitioner with a lecturer, supervisor, mentor or peers to gain direction for future learning or development, all of the portfolio requirements and guidelines as well as feedback processes and details need to be focused towards this end. Alternatively, if the purpose of the assessment is to provide a summative (final) judgement about performance or achievement, then the associated achievement criteria should be clear in the assessment guidelines/rubric/feedback sheet. In addition to the traditional notions of assessment, portfolios may also be used as part of an institution's audit system as a cluster of data to evaluate the institution's success in supporting student and staff performance outcomes. In this way, information generated through assessment of individual portfolios can inform the development and review of relevant policies, guidelines and criteria, including the need for staff development. To take advantage of these opportunities, however, and ensure that assessment practices do achieve the intended outcomes of supporting learning and/or ascertaining the achievement of performance criteria, quality assessment design is an imperative.

While this chapter has been written for current and future assessors of portfolios, people compiling their own portfolio will also benefit from understanding the perspective of the assessor when preparing their portfolio or reviewing the assessment feedback. The chapter includes an overview of portfolio assessment and evaluation, as this understanding is necessary to inform the design of quality assessment processes that stimulate learning and quality reporting mechanisms. The section entitled 'Designing an assessment rubric' has been included to assist in developing a comprehensive feedback summary sheet to assist both the assessor and the student/applicant. Various other exemplars and activities have also been included to assist the reader in applying these principles to practice.

Basic assumptions about assessment

As students, we generally assume that our work is marked or assessed purely for the purposes of awarding a grade and providing us with feedback. As part of this understanding, we are aware that our work will be graded either in comparison to other students' work (norm-referenced) or against a set of criteria (criterion-referenced). While it is true that a large component of assessment is the ascertaining of a student's performance level, it is important to note that good assessment can do so much more than this. Arguably, assessment is the conduit between teaching and learning, in that

information can be made available but a student only really learns through applying this knowledge to practice and receiving feedback about their performance (Wiliam 2013). Further to this, timely assessment can provide educators and administrators with important information to refine the direction of educational delivery to better support students' learning. Additionally, quality assessment can stimulate and direct students' learning and performance, giving them incentive and direction on how to perform well (Wiliam 2013). In order to achieve this, assessments need to be well structured and timely. The instructions and assessment criteria should be freely available to the students, as these can potentially provide the stimulus for students to extend their achievements. The students should have a solid understanding of the criteria for performance, plus the necessary tools/support to achieve the desired outcome. While it is now standard practice to provide students with assessment criteria, often there is inadequate time and resources given to assist them to understand the criteria and how it is to be applied (Wiliam 2013). Furthermore, as educationalists, we often underestimate the requisite skills needed to achieve the assessment outcome. As this chapter will reiterate, designing and executing a quality assessment item requires each of these components to be considered.

Portfolio approaches and the impact on assessment

The use of portfolios as a reputable form of assessing and developing professional practice is now well established (Haldane 2014). However, it is important that it not be assumed that there is a single appropriate approach to portfolio assessment. The portfolio approach will impact significantly on the manner in which the assessment needs to be managed. A portfolio is both process- and product-oriented. A process-oriented approach is a formative, educative and process-driven approach that highlights the processes of recording, mapping and moving towards personalised professional or practice development goals. The 'product-' or 'achievement-oriented' approach is about demonstrating the achievement of a standard for the purposes of accreditation, promotion or gaining recognition of an accomplishment of some kind. Assessment processes need to reflect the different purposes of a portfolio in order to inform and support the student/

staff member in achieving and being rewarded for the intended outcome.

For the process-oriented dimension of a portfolio, assessment needs to reward successful use of reflection, critical evaluation and soundness of planning. As will be elaborated upon later in this chapter, assessment rubrics and other forms of feedback frameworks are useful in making these sorts of achievement components apparent to the learner and providing a focus for feedback. Associated with this, the ongoing (formative) or final (summative) feedback should be learning-focused and hence provide explanations of learning processes, relevant inspirational examples and direction to resources. This form of feedback is usually a cyclical, ongoing process where advice and feedback are given over time with the intention of continued growth and development. Peer feedback may be appropriate in situations such as this, as its reciprocal nature can enhance the understandings of both those receiving and giving the feedback.

Assessment of outcomes is required for a product/achievement dimension of a portfolio. As a consequence, the assessment framework needs to provide a clear reference to the performance standards being assessed and the criteria being used to make the final judgement. Feedback may include direction for continued improvement but, importantly, needs to clarify the basis of the final decision regarding success or otherwise of attaining the required outcome. Both those being assessed and those auditing the assessors need to be able to see how a judgement, grade or other decision was arrived at. Prescribed requirements, such as those written by regulatory authorities or professional organisations, need to be evident within the assessment criteria and feedback provided. Promotion applications or applications to the regulatory authority – for instance, for advanced practice status – are primarily 'product-oriented' portfolios.

As we have indicated, most portfolios require description and evidence of both processes and outcomes and so dichotomous comparison between 'process' and 'product' portfolios is mostly not apparent in practice. Students being supported to develop their professional portfolios are useful examples of where a blended feedback approach is required, whereby a combination of feedback about ongoing learning and development, plus comment on the quality of the product outcomes,

is necessary. It is useful, however, to consider first the two extremes of portfolio styles as a way of better understanding portfolio dimensions and the related assessment criteria. Table 6.1 highlights the two extremes of portfolio style and the different ways that purpose, structure and assessment may be approached in each of these. A blended approach may use components of each, but this needs to be worked through carefully to avoid contradiction and unnecessary complexity.

SUMMARY POINTS

- Assessment is central to learning, as it enables students to apply their understanding to practice in a guided and supported manner.
- The central tenet in the assessment of the educational or learning portfolio dimension is to support and direct continuous improvement, and in doing so support and reward the processes of self-assessment, reflection, planning and implementation.
- The central tenet in the assessment of the product/achievement portfolio dimension is to support and reward the framing of a claim that is substantiated with sufficient quality evidence.

Portfolio assessment and evaluation

While the terms 'assessment' and 'evaluation' are commonly used interchangeably, particularly in the professional practice context, their meaning in the professional/educational setting is not necessarily the same. In this context, evaluation generally describes the broader process of institutional appraisal and feedback, whereas assessment pertains to the learning/performance outcomes of the individual. A rather simplistic definition would be that a student or staff member's portfolio is assessed, while an organisation's performance is evaluated. The relevance of this definition within this text is that the assessment of individual portfolios can be useful in informing the institution's evaluation processes. While this chapter will mostly

TABLE 6.1

Two professional portfolio approaches

	Process-oriented	Product-oriented
Portfolio purpose	Development/continuous improvement through reflective practice Intended to enable learners to monitor and reflect on their learning and present a coherent systematic account. Promotes student and/or health professional self-assessment and development across specified areas of knowledge, skills and attitudes. May include what has occurred in the building of the portfolio, including reflective aspects of self-assessment, planning and progress. Records and reflections of interactions related to the stages, journey or development of student/staff learning. Progress is a strong element.	Demonstration of achievement outcomes Makes a particular and definitive argument or case for achievement, usually for certification or re-certification of licence to practise, for promotion, or for recognition of prior learning (RPL). The focus is on an end-product that demonstrates the best-possible argument, case or presentation of the necessary level of performance or achievement against a set standard.
Portfolio structure and organisation, including evidence types and use	Personalised structure, chronological substructure Structure can vary, with portfolio authors potentially choosing an approach and the materials for inclusion that best support their learning. Because the purpose of this portfolio dimension is to demonstrate learning over time, a chronological substructure is commonly used whereby earlier entries provide the basis for reflection on the growth made.	Prescribed thematic structure The portfolio is organised according to a clear, prescribed structure that may be criteria, standards and/or outcomes, as prescribed by the institution being 'applied' to. Includes documents demonstrating work-related performance outcomes. Ideally, the description of the achievement of performance outcomes will be benchmarked against best-practice standards.

Continued

TABLE 6.1

Two professional portfolio approaches—cont'd

	Process-oriented	Product-oriented
Portfolio assessment	Integrated or holistic The purpose of this assessment is to engage the author for the purposes of continuous improvement. Formative or ongoing assessment is common and may or may not result in a final/formal assessment judgement/grade. For grading purposes, the complete collection of materials or record of development is assessed against the author's claims of self-understanding and professional development. Assessment criteria are focused on the author's ability to assess a situation, critically reflect, plan, effect change and evaluate outcomes. In addition to providing recognition of the quality learning processed, feedback should also include direction and resources for continued learning.	Methodological or systematic The purpose of the assessment is to ensure that a set standard is met, particularly in the case of accreditation, promotion and RPL. The assessor is accountable to the institution to ensure compliance with these prescribed standards, and therefore will draw on these and broader notions of 'in the public/institution's interest' to make their decision. Therefore, issues of patient and public safety must be clearly attended to. The portfolio is assessed systematically according to criteria (criterion-referenced assessment) such as educational, statutory, professional or organisational standards or outcomes. Feedback should clarify and justify the assessment decisions, the detail of which can be called upon if the results are audited.

address the assessment in education, it is important to consider how staff or student portfolios could provide useful data to inform healthcare and educational institutions' evaluation of their own performance. It would, of course, be appropriate that staff and students were made aware if this were to be instituted, and systems of anonymity and data management (as per other quality control measures) utilised.

Why assess?

While there is a range of reasons why educational providers, employing organisations and regulators might use assessment processes, these can generally be reduced to two broad and potentially overlapping categories – namely, to:

- direct and stimulate student/staff/applicant learning, including self-understanding
- regulate/accredit/communicate professional/ educational standards (Hallam et al. 2010).

As previously discussed, both of these purposes influence the way in which assessments are designed and what criteria are used to pass judgement on the outcomes. While it is essential for the assessor to understand this if they are to provide high-quality, rigorous and consistent assessment processes, it is also useful for the learner/ applicant to understand the perspective of the assessor. The following activity is designed to support both the assessor and the person being assessed to understand the range of learning and performance outcomes that might be developed and assessed via a portfolio.

ACTIVITY: INTENDED PORTFOLIO OUTCOMES

Table 6.2 has been constructed in a format that you can reproduce and complete using your own learning priorities and ideas. The aim is for you to consider a range of intended learning outcomes for both learning/process and achievement/product portfolios dimensions. To achieve this, you will need to list the different portfolio activities that you are aware of, and then:

1 consider which of these involves a learning process or achievement outcome

2 list each within the appropriate column.

To assist, examples have been included in the table.

TABLE 6.2
Intended portfolio outcomes

Purpose: Demonstrating learning process	Purpose: Demonstrating product achievement
Example: Learning processes: • identifying personal learning needs in relation to leadership, clinical experience, change agent, communication • developing a learning plan • maintaining records about the plan implementation, including reflecting upon the impact of the various learning experiences.	Example: Evidence of performance outcomes relating to: • leadership • clinical expertise • change agent • communication skills.

Assessing to direct and stimulate learning

What and how students learn is determined to a significant extent by how they perceive the assessment requirements (Biggs & Tang 2011). From a learner's perspective, assessment requirements become the focus of learning (Jessop 2017). In doing so, assessment provides the incentive and direction for student learning. Process skills such as teamwork (including inter-professional practice), communication and critical thinking can be developed and refined while developing an assessment product such as a poster presentation, essay or staff development presentation. Quality assessment activities that reward the learner for using solid learning processes and meeting quality outcomes have the potential to position the learner for lifelong learning that supports the application of knowledge to practice. This, however,

is the greatest of educational challenges within the environment of 'time-poor' students. If assessments are overly onerous, students will resent the time needed to complete them and look for shortcuts. This has the potential to create a sense of separateness, both between theory and practice and between students and staff. It is therefore important that staff work closely with students to support them through the process and reiterate the professional relevance of the task.

Portfolios are frequently used in education of health professionals as learning activities and assessment items (Buckley et al. 2010, Green et al. 2014, Haldane 2014). As has been identified, complex activities such as assembling a portfolio, especially if laden with new technology-related skills, has the potential to be problematic for students (Gadbury-Amyot &

Overman 2018). In their eagerness to teach new skills and understandings, educators (including those in staff development) often 'frontload' learning experiences with terminology and theory frameworks, rather than engaging the students/staff in activities that would support progressive skill acquisition. Many of us will have experienced this in our early exposure to theoretical frameworks, research methodology and critical thinking. Unless done well, the teaching and assessment of these often conceptual topics can result in students failing to meet the deep and applied learning outcomes intended. It is important that the designers of assessment items think about this and design assessments in association with educational support that will enable the intended learning outcomes.

Portfolio development has been identified as influential in developing student and staff abilities. A 2010 study of the types of portfolio, particularly e-portfolios, that were in use in Australian higher education found that 'ePortfolios had the potential to assist students [to] become reflective learners, conscious of their personal and professional strengths and weaknesses, as well as to make their existing and developing skills more explicit…' (Hallam et al. 2010, p. 1). These outcomes, however, are achieved only if integrated into a broader curriculum or institutional system that supports progressive student or staff development in a range of associated knowledge, skills and attitudes. It is important to remind ourselves that a single assessment item rarely has a significant and ongoing influence on learning and performance outcomes. Rather, learning is progressive, cumulative and responsive to the broader cultural environment, such that in addition to providing quality assessment support it is also important to have a learning culture that supports openness and rewards genuine achievements.

Following on from this sentiment, the large and complex nature of compiling a portfolio means that this exercise is best undertaken progressively over time, with a tolerance of developing ideas and achievements. The challenge for the educator is to design a program of study and assessment that will support the requisite skills and understandings without distorting student or staff learning such that irrelevant or superficial learning takes precedence over genuine and effective outcomes. Learning can be distorted, for example, if portfolio users

are overly distracted by the technology or terminology used to explain aspects of the portfolio, and this becomes learning at the expense of the intended learning outcomes, including reflective learning or understanding of personal competence. Similar issues occur, for example, when the technical/formatting aspects of referencing are taught in a manner that distracts students from understanding the need to evaluate sourced information for relevance and quality. Of concern is that if portfolio users do not see the value of compiling a portfolio, or of framing their arguments, there is a risk that the exercise will be interpreted as rhetorical, burdensome, and of little benefit to professional practice.

As identified above, it is important to be cognisant of both the intended and unintended learning outcomes that may result from any assessment item. Designing quality assessment experiences requires that students are provided with learning supports and opportunities that will enhance their understanding and skills in achieving this intended student learning.

Early in an individual's professional development, detailed directions for portfolio development may help guide their learning activities; this may be reduced later in the program when the objective is for students or applicants to demonstrate initiative and self-direction. For this reason, for example, direction given to nurse practitioner applicants in developing their portfolios may be deliberately broad, because the ability to evaluate and assimilate a range of materials in order to develop and substantiate an original argument would be considered integral to the performance requirements at that level. If this is the objective, then in addition to informing the applicants of what is expected, the assessment process needs to reward the achievement of this outcome. In some instances, the reward will be a higher grade; in other cases, such as for the nurse practitioner applicant, the demonstration of higher-level analysis is a requirement for professional entry.

Assessing outcomes in a portfolio

Ensuring that students or applicants meet a required standard is a central tenet of any educational or employment assessment. The 'gatekeeping' role of regulators, educationalists and employers is central to their particular purpose. Similarly, students, staff members and applicants need to receive recognition of their achievements because this will motivate future learning and development.

A portfolio must be made up of evidence of sufficient quality. This means that the evidence items within the portfolio need to:

- demonstrate contemporary practice
- contain a reflective or evaluative component
- attend to the standard/competency identified
- be validated by others.

Further, the items of evidence need to form a cohesive whole that supports the claim/argument of competence. In order to ensure that this is achieved, concepts of quality and wholeness must be reflected in assessment instructions and then again in the grading/assessment criteria.

In short, the need to direct, encourage and reward specific outcomes will shape the way in which you design and communicate the assessment process. The questions you may wish to ask yourself are:

- What do you want to assess (the content of the portfolio – namely, items of evidence and/or the demonstrated process of compiling and justifying a portfolio)?
- How should the assessment objectives and process be communicated to the applicant/student?
- How will assessment rigour, validity and reliability be met?

Your answers to these questions will influence the assessment process you develop. Later sections of this chapter will further assist you in this process.

What is to be assessed?

As with any assessment process, it is important to clarify from the outset what is being assessed (assessment/learning objectives) and how it is to be evaluated (assessment/feedback schema). Pay considerable attention to this in the assessment design stages. Portfolios can be used to support learning and assess any number of outcomes, including demonstrating self-determination through:

- reflecting upon and framing a claim of competence/achievement
- substantiating a claim using a range of quality evidence
- assessing personal learning needs
- developing relevant learning and career plans
- evaluating the success of achievements.

'Producing a portfolio' is not necessarily in itself a learning objective; rather, the portfolio is often a tool to achieve a more specific objective, such as one of those listed above.

For the purposes of the remainder of this section, it will be assumed that the broad objectives of what is to be assessed have been set. In some cases, these will be learning objectives accompanied by detailed assessment instructions. In other instances, such as promotion or position applications, the applicant will need to interpret these through reflecting on the task required. It is important to understand, when developing a portfolio for these types of applications, that the applicant is being

---

SUMMARY POINTS

- Portfolios may be used as assessment items to direct learning and provide recognition of achievement.
- In addition to providing an assessment opportunity, staff and student portfolios contain potentially useful evaluation data to gauge the institution's success in supporting student and staff performance outcomes.
- While assessment is a major driver of learning, importantly this may include quality (deep, applied and intended) learning, or unintended learning such as surface learning and attitudinal development that impairs future learning.
- Assessments should support and reward well-framed and appropriate claims that are adequately supported by quality, diverse and verifiable evidence.

assessed on their ability to independently argue their case; hence, detailed instructions may well be limited.

Whatever the situation, it is important to consider the overall 'intent' of the assessment/portfolio requirement throughout the assembly and assessment process, because this will help you to clarify the priorities that should be explicit in both the portfolio and the assessment feedback framework.

As the following information will detail, the learning objectives and broader intended learning outcomes will inform the appropriateness of grading structures and assessment feedback schemas.

Awarding grades

The following discussion pertains to the assessment processes associated with awarding grades – namely, norm-referenced grades and criterion-referenced grades. Norm-referenced grades for assessments are distributed according to a predetermined distribution across the candidate population. Grades are attributed according to the students' comparative rankings (Chan 2014). Criterion-referenced grades, on the other hand, are awarded according to a set of predetermined criteria. If, for example, all students performed at the required level for a distinction, based on the criteria, they could all receive a distinction grade. This could not happen in norm-referenced grading.

Criterion-referenced grading can also apply to 'non-graded pass/fail', an alternative form of assessment grading. This approach is often used in instances where a range of higher-level achievements cannot be reliably or easily assessed, and so an outcome of 'achieved' or 'not achieved' is most appropriate. This is not to say that the assessment is less rigorous; on the contrary, pass marks may be as high as 100%, because an underlying premise of criterion-referenced assessment is that the pass criteria reflect the minimum standard of practice required. Pass/fail criterion-referenced grading is usually used for assessing technical skills where the requirement is that the applicant meets a minimum level of performance, such as proficiency in performing cardiopulmonary resuscitation. Similarly, criterion-referenced pass/fail grading is often used when evaluating portfolios for regulation and promotion purposes, because it is both

irrelevant and difficult to ascertain qualitative differences beyond the required 'acceptable level of performance'.

In the educational setting, however, non-graded assessment outcomes are problematic because the merit of the student's performance is not communicated to the student or in their academic record.

Academic records and associated calculations such as mean/average grades are used often as the initial screening process for employers and educational institutions. It is therefore important that grades awarded to students reflect the range of their achievements, and are not limited to learning outcomes that are traditionally accepted as 'easier to grade'.

Having identified whether normative or criterion-referenced grading is to be used, it is necessary to develop a marking or assessment schema. It is imperative that the assessment criteria are designed to evaluate the learning/assessment objectives identified and that they are clearly understood by those involved. The concepts that have been identified as the 'criteria of quality' will also inform the grading details of the schema. For instance, earlier in this book we referred to indicators of quality evidence as items that are current, relate to contemporary practice and demonstrate the performance outcomes relevant to the competency/standard in question. It is important to have the indicators of quality inform the design of a scoring schema or rubric, so that the pre-established criteria against which the student's or applicant's work is to be evaluated are clearly detailed.

What is an assessment rubric?

An assessment rubric is in effect the criteria that explains grading standards (Biggs & Tang 2011). A rubric is required for each assessment item. These rubrics are sometimes called 'grading schemes', 'scoring guides' or 'feedback sheets'. Rubrics can assess processes, such as psychomotor skills, or products such as essays. They may be analytic or holistic, general or task-specific (Brookhart 2013). The format of a rubric can vary, but typically it is in the form of a table that includes:

- a rating scale against which either the components of the product or the product as a whole are judged (header row)

- a list of assignment components or objectives that are being assessed (column 1)
- individual cells detailing the corresponding level of performance for the grade awarded.

Table 6.3 provides a brief summary of these components.

Table 6.4 is a more complete assessment rubric that demonstrates the application of these components. This kind of rubric would be commonly used in the higher education sector. The first column details one component of the assessment task. The top/header row of the table sets out the five-level scoring criteria. As shown in this example, the range of grades is not necessarily a consequence of the frequency of behaviours; rather, qualitative increments are added to the aggregation of content. The qualitative increments shown in the table have been informed by the work of Biggs and Tang (2011). It is important that the scoring criteria used reflect the institutional policies and grading schemas such that all parties can see how the final grade has been awarded. It is important to note that students and auditors alike should be able to see a direct relationship between the feedback provided within the assessment rubric and the final grade. For this to be possible, the rubric must be clear from the perspective of both. The use of complex language in rubrics has been reported as a source of confusion for students who also may not know the most effective way to read a rubric (Colvin et al. 2016).

As you will note from the example in Table 6.4, even at this level of detail some interpretation is required. It is important that this interpretation be made clear to students, as described later in this chapter in the section 'Ways to support student learning through assessment'. Furthermore, it is essential that all staff assisting and marking students' work have a consistent and applied understanding of the rubric. This will also be covered later when we discuss the moderation processes in the section on validity and reliability of assessment.

Student/applicant feedback

As demonstrated in Table 6.4, it is possible to provide a significant amount of information to students, staff and applicants about the assessment process. It is now expected that if quality teaching practices are being used, assessment processes and information should be provided to students/applicants well in advance, with many educational organisations providing grading schemas as part of the assignment instructions. Complex tasks such as the assembling of a portfolio require additional support; students and applicants gain considerable assistance from discussions with those who will be evaluating their portfolios (Scholes et al. 2004). The inclusion of a formative assessment process, whereby feedback and direction are provided part-way through an assessment activity, is particularly important for large and complex assessment activities such as portfolio submissions (Jasper & Fulton 2005). These feedback comments may be embedded within the text of the assessment activity and/or presented as a written/verbal summary.

The nature and extent of feedback comments are generally dependent upon the time and resources available, and the purpose of the assessment. In formative assessment situations, where students and applicants may

TABLE 6.3
Assessment rubric

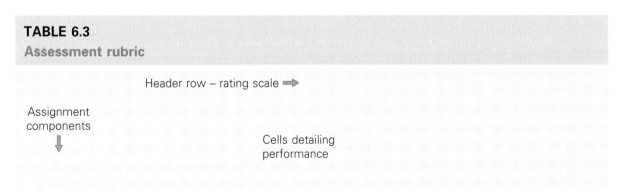

TABLE 6.4

Example: Student assignment assessment rubric assessment item: Nurse practitioner portfolio submission (Master's Program)

Assessment components	Advanced (score range 85–100%) The learner is able to demonstrate extension beyond 'proficient' to include insightful questioning and development of hypotheses and theories	Proficient (65–84%) The learner offers an integrated understanding of all essential aspects, such that the whole has coherent structure and meaning	Functional (55–64%) The learner focuses on the relevant area and works appropriately with all the essential aspects. The learner provides correct materials with discrete and separate items of information	Developing (minimal pass) (50–54%) The learner focuses on the relevant area but requires direction in some non-essential aspects	Unsatisfactory (0–49%) The learner is engaged in the task, but is distracted or misled by irrelevant aspects
Translates and integrates evidence into planning care	Has demonstrated 'proficient' criteria, plus has used extensive quality literature to effectively support emerging trends. Included high-level critique of research when explaining relevance to own practice environment. Original and creative thinking demonstrated through the quality of own publications and presentations.	Has demonstrated the use of critical, reflective thinking to synthesise a sound argument that this standard is met. Has provided relevant and contemporary evidence to substantiate claims. Evidence consistently supported by research literature, including evidence from other disciplines to inform and/or initiate change in educational, clinical or organisational decisions described.	Has applied relevant evidence of the use of research and/or the integration of current research findings into practice; however, the discussion did not completely articulate how research influenced or initiated change in educational, clinical or organisational decision making.	Predominantly sound understanding of research applied to practice, with occasional confusing explanations of how this is being achieved. Has drawn on several relevant items of research to inform practice, including systematic reviews. While has omitted to draw on all relevant research, has shown the ability to utilise evidence to inform own practice if able. Needs to develop strategies on how to stay abreast of contemporary research findings. Is using research to inform some but not all educational, clinical or organisational decisions described.	Has not provided sufficient evidence of the use of research methods or the integration of research findings to inform or initiate a change in educational, clinical or organisational decision-making. May have used relevant references, but failed to critique and apply information adequately.

Has demonstrated a conscious and deliberate mechanism to ethically explore therapeutic options, including consistently high standard of integration of assessment information, the person's informed decision and best-available evidence.

Has shown the ability to utilise evidence to inform own practice, though the explanations of how this was achieved may have omissions. Is using research to inform a majority of educational, clinical or organisational decisions described. Has clear understanding of and strategies to address the above deficits. Has demonstrated a conscious and deliberate mechanism to ethically explore therapeutic options, including integration of assessment information, the person's informed decision and best-available evidence.

Has demonstrated an understanding of mechanisms to ethically explore therapeutic options, but has applied these inconsistently. Is aware of their limitations in this area and has a strategy for achieving this shortfall.

May be providing safe care, but reliant on others to inform and/or initiate change in educational, clinical or organisational decisions described. May have attempted to demonstrate mechanisms used to ethically explore therapeutic options, but no evidence that this is consistently integrated in practice.

use feedback to improve upon the assessment activity, the feedback needs to provide both direction and rationale for action. The inclusion of both broad and detailed direction, plus links to resources and explanations using exemplars to demonstrate the applications of principles, are useful strategies to achieve this. Within summative assessment situations, in addition to formative feedback, it is also important that clarification be provided about the basis of the final decision or grade. Statements that demonstrate the alignment between performance aspects of the portfolio and the assessment grading criteria are useful to help the applicant/student understand how and why the final grade/decision was awarded. It is just as important for the student/applicant to understand why they were successful as it is to understand what else could be achieved.

In both summative and formative assessment situations, the feedback needs to reflect the intent of the assessment, and therefore must include comment about the holistic direction of the assignment, rather than overly emphasising specific components such as editorial changes.

Ways to support student learning through assessment

The following is a quick catch-up on the importance of having students/applicants understand the assessment criteria described above. All too often, assessment rubrics or other performance measures are provided to students and applicants as if this is all they need to be able to do to focus their achievements. Unfortunately, this is sometimes creating unanticipated confusion rather than clarity.

Assessment feedback needs to be timely in order to be effective in stimulating learning. No doubt we can all relate to the disappointment of receiving a poorer assignment grade than we anticipated and having no opportunity to make restitution. Well-designed assessment items that enable us to have early feedback that facilitate remedial action are clearly a more ideal outcome in supporting learning. As a consequence, most educational institutions now use early assessment items with this very intention. While there are many ways to do this, a useful approach is to break a large assessment

item into parts, and have students submit components such as the literature review, a single section or the overall plan for their first assignment. This approach both encourages the students to manage their time well, while also enabling them to receive feedback to direct their next assignments. Therefore, if you are designing a portfolio assessment for your students, consider what early assessment would best assist in their success. A combination of completing a single clinical competency/ standard section, plus a list of the items of evidence that might be used as appendices, is a useful approach. Depending on your class structure, this may also be done as a group assessment or class activity.

It is essential that you spend time ensuring that students understand the performance requirements. There is no need for secrets when it comes to assessments. Students should be given every opportunity to achieve well, and hence should understand what is expected of them. While it is now usual to make assessment rubrics/ marking guides available to students, it is less common to spend time ensuring that they understand what these criteria mean. Given that many of the concepts and performance indicators are complex, it is little wonder that students often don't understand the assessment performance criteria. Concepts such as 'scholarly critique' and 'supporting arguments with high-level evidence' can be difficult for students to grasp. The following are a few ideas for classroom/online activities to assist students to understand the performance criteria of assessment items:

- Have students collaborate in designing the assessment rubric. Provide a rubric for students to critique. Encourage them to ask questions and suggest changes. There will be times when students will need to consider the full range of performance categories and the measure of how these are achieved. If, however, the performance categories are already largely known – for instance, these are the professional standards or promotion criteria – have the students work in groups to develop the levels of performance for each.
- Provide examples and exemplars of work, and include rubric-based discussions as to the quality of these items (Jones et al. 2017). This is a very useful class exercise, as it can generate considerable discussion about what constitutes a quality product.

- Have individual students develop an early assessment item that is then anonymously reviewed by a peer in class (Jones et al. 2017). Having students mark a draft or component of their peers' work in class is another way of having them consider what makes some work good and other work merely average.

Clearly, you will need to design a strategy that best suits your students' needs; however, do not underestimate the need for some intervention to assist students to understand the application of your marking guide.

Validity and reliability of assessment

Ensuring both validity (assessing what is intended and not something else) and reliability (consistency within the assessment process and between assessors) is clearly of concern when assessing portfolios (Gadbury-Amyot et al. 2014, Haldane 2014). As has been discussed earlier, poorly designed assessment activities, or a lack of learning resources to support an outcome, can mean that assessment items distract from, rather than support, student/staff learning. This lack of validity has been observed when technical processes associated with e-portfolios, for example, override the intended learning. Similarly, assessment outcomes should be consistent, such that the process is fair and reliable, no matter who is the assessor.

As a consequence of the need for reliability and protection against plagiarism, the assessment process may include further verification such as referees' reports or a presentation/'portfolio defence' requirement. A 'portfolio defence' is where an applicant provides a presentation exemplifying aspects of their portfolio and is available to respond to questions. This was a common requirement for nurse practitioner application processes, for example, prior to the introduction and availability of accredited programs of study. In some respects, a job interview is also a form of portfolio defence.

To a large extent, assessment validity and reliability can be maintained through the design and formulation of a clear grading schema (Biggs & Tang 2011). The reliability of an assessment schema can be enhanced by moderation, where there is more than one assessor.

There is a degree of professional judgement involved in any assessment process. It is therefore important that those people grading the portfolios share a clear understanding of the aims of the portfolio and assessment criteria.

By now you will recognise that portfolios have a place in the assessment of learning as part of educational programs, organisational performance reviews and individual career planning. The assessment of a portfolio is clearly linked to the portfolio purpose, regardless of whether the portfolio is for an individual seeking to enact a career pathway or an educator, regulator or employer using portfolios to stimulate learning and make judgements about individual suitability. We have discussed the relevance of incremental merit-based grades and criterion-referenced assessment, and applied these to grading rubrics and checklists. Integral to the message of this chapter is the responsibility of the assessor to design assessment processes that positively influence learning outcomes and are fair.

The information covered in this chapter is reinforced by the comments in the Practice Exemplar below from Jean Gilmour, an experienced assessor of portfolios across academic and regulatory contexts.

Conclusion

This chapter has provided an overview of practices and principles related to portfolio assessment to support the development of quality practice. It has been long understood that learning is related to experience. Student learning is often driven by assessment, with rewards evident as grades and recognition; as a consequence, students engage with learning tasks when the relationship between these tasks and their assessment is apparent. To achieve the intended learning, however, assessments need to be designed in a manner that supports the achievement of quality learning outcomes. Assessment guidelines and requirements that are confusing, overly laden with technological or other distractors, or do not relate to the students' perceptions of 'real-world

PRACTICE EXEMPLAR

Jean Gilmour, a senior lecturer in the School of Health Sciences at Massey University (New Zealand), has been involved in assessing nurse practitioner applicants. Jean has provided the following practice exemplar:

Assessing portfolios is a complex task. Therefore, think carefully about how best to communicate effectively your competence and professional contributions to the portfolio reviewer. A scholarly, fit-for-purpose and well-structured portfolio is a powerful communication tool for showcasing your practice and your ability.

Some specific strategies to consider when developing a portfolio are as follows:

- Gather evidence as the opportunities arise, even if you are not planning on applying for an advanced practice role. Aspirations change and grow as your career progresses. Substantial evidence developed over a sustained time period is required to demonstrate practice at advanced levels.
- When gathering evidence be mindful of confidentiality obligations and abide by organisational policies. Oversights in these areas can lead to questions around professional conduct.
- Take the time to review relevant standards/competencies carefully and make sure you understand the level/ scope of practice required to meet them. Producing evidence demonstrating a less advanced stage of practice will disadvantage you.
- Make sure your evidence is clearly linked to the relevant competency/standard. Do not put the reviewer in the position of having to guess why a piece of evidence might have been included.
- Engage in peer-review processes and mentoring arrangements with your colleagues during portfolio development. Critique of your evidence will challenge your assumptions and expand your practice horizons.
- Take care to demonstrate that your practice is culturally safe. Evidence of cultural safety includes demonstrating your ability to be reflexive about the values and practices of your own culture and health service culture, along with the impact of those values and practices on the options and perceptions of the people using the health services. Case studies and practice accounts illustrating culturally safe practice, verified by an appropriate person such as the person receiving care and/or a culturally appropriate third party, are important sources of evidence.

SUMMARY POINTS

- Portfolios can be used to support learning and assess any number of outcomes that align with personal and professional self-determination.
- The purpose of awarding grades is to communicate achievements succinctly.
- Criterion-referenced grades awarded to portfolios may be incremental merit-based grades (e.g. fail through to distinction), or binary grades (e.g. pass/fail) or a combination of both using assessment hurdles within incremental merit-based grading systems.
- The grading approach used should reflect the purpose of the assessment.
- Scoring rubrics are widely used by assessors to grade complex tasks such as portfolios.
- Feedback needs to support the intent of the assessment – namely, to provide incentive and skills for further learning and/or to understand the basis of the achievement being recognised.
- Collaboration between team members and other assessors is required to support valid (assess what is being intended) and reliable (consistently applied) assessment.

practice' can result in negative learning. In these scenarios, students might fail to learn and develop the skills that were intended, or – possibly worse – develop negative attitudes to learning and change. In addition to providing assignment instructions that are clear and are associated with supportive learning resources, assessment feedback schemas need also to support intended learning outcomes. Assessment grading and feedback should be a transparent exercise whereby the learner is provided with sufficient information and incentive to allow them to understand what is required to achieve a superior product. Assessment feedback schemas and rubrics are routinely provided as part of assignment instructions. Importantly, students and others submitting their work to be assessed need to understand what these schemas mean in order to benefit from this information. This chapter has provided this level of information so that the rationales and approaches within assessment design and implementation can be understood by all participants in the assessment process.

Chapter 7

Examples of health practitioners' approaches to planning and evaluating CPD

Introduction

The aim of this book is to guide health practitioners in understanding how to develop and present a portfolio that demonstrates their professional efforts, progress and capabilities. Employers and regulatory authorities require individual practitioners to continue learning after entry to practice in order to achieve continuing safe healthcare. This responsibility of practitioners includes keeping sufficient evidence of quality practice and performance.

This final chapter provides some practical examples of the approaches different health practitioners might take in developing their professional portfolio in the following roles:

- midwifery (contribution from Sara Bayes)
- registered nursing (contribution from Lisa Devey)
- enrolled nursing (contribution from Síobhán Bidgood)
- occupational therapy (contribution from Sue Gilbert-Hunt)
- paramedicine (contribution from Joe Acker)
- pharmacy (contribution from Kearney Gleadhill).

Each of the above health practitioners has provided an exemplar of how they use portfolios within their continuing professional development. While there has been some updating for this edition of the text, editing of submissions to assist in readability and reduce repetition of information, variation remains where it is necessary to provide relevant background for individual professional groups.

The Australian Health Practitioner Regulation Agency (AHPRA) and each of the National Boards implement the National Registration and Accreditation Scheme through a nationally consistent approach to registration standards, guidelines and auditing health practitioners' compliance with the mandatory standards, which includes a continuing professional development standard. (For details of these various standards, codes and guidelines, including the audit process, see the relevant National Board's website.)

The continuing professional development standards detailed by each of the National Boards stipulate the ongoing requirements for each of the registered health professions, including the number of development hours and types of documentation required. Some Boards provide an example template to meet the needs of their audit process. The audit involves the Boards randomly identifying a sample of registered health professionals throughout the year and conducting a structured process through which those selected need to provide evidence to support their declaration that they have met the registration standards for the profession. This book promotes a more comprehensive and ongoing portfolio process through which evidence of professional ability is generated and updated to serve a variety of career purposes, which may include supplying evidence for audit requirements.

The discussion below is designed to supplement details on portfolio development provided earlier in this book. Each section in the chapter highlights the requirements of continuing professional development and provides examples for different disciplines. Although each section refers to one area of health practitioner practice, the descriptions and examples of how to reflect on, describe and document practice may be of value to other health practitioners. Standards, guidelines and policy will change over time, so it is also strongly recommended that the websites of the National Boards be accessed for current and updated details about the specific requirements of continuing professional development standards.

Communicating competence for midwives, registered nurses and enrolled nurses

'Midwife', 'registered nurse', 'enrolled nurse' and 'nurse practitioner' are titles protected by law, and anyone using these titles is regulated by the Nursing and Midwifery Board of Australia (NMBA). Continuing professional development is a requirement of registration for these practitioners and is defined by the NMBA as 'the means by which members of the profession maintain, improve and broaden their knowledge, expertise and competence, and develop the personal and professional qualities required throughout their professional lives' (Nursing and Midwifery Board of Australia 2016c). In addition to the continuing professional development standard, the NMBA website has guidelines for continuing professional development.

As discussed in the earlier chapters of this book, continuing professional development is conducted in a cycle that involves reviewing and documenting one's practice, identifying one's learning needs, planning and participating in relevant learning activities, and reflecting on the value of those activities. Practice is defined by the NMBA in a way that recognises more than clinical care (Nursing and Midwifery Board of Australia 2016a).

The current continuing professional development requirements are for documentation of continuing professional development to include dates, a brief description of the outcomes, and the number of hours spent on each activity. All evidence must be verified and must demonstrate that the registered individual has:

- identified and prioritised their learning needs based on an evaluation of their practice against the relevant competency or professional practice standards (in this case, the practice standards for midwives, registered nurses, enrolled nurses and nurse practitioners)
- developed a learning plan based on identified learning needs
- participated in effective learning activities relevant to their learning needs
- reflected on the value of the learning activities or the effect that participation will have on their practice.

The NMBA provides on its website a list of *suggested* continuing professional development activities. (See https://www.nursingmidwiferyboard.gov.au/Codes-Guidelines-Statements/FAQ/CPD-FAQ-for-nurses-and-midwives.aspx.)

The NMBA also provides a number of useful web-based resources for continuing professional development, including a template document in which the activities of the continuing professional development cycle can be recorded. (These resources can be found at www.nursingmidwiferyboard.gov.au/Registration-and-Endorsement/Audit.aspx.)

Communicating Competence for Midwifery Practice

Sara Bayes

Midwives in Australia are employed in a wide range of roles. Some roles require the application of the entire range of fundamental midwifery knowledge and skills, while in others the midwife uses only some aspects of their practice. Midwives' professional development must be directly related to their practice context and knowledge deficits. The continuing professional development plan that each midwife develops will be different from those of their colleagues.

It is essential to examine both the current learning needs and any future career ambitions so that skills and knowledge deficits relative to each can be determined and planned for. Jenny (see Example 7.1) has identified that she greatly enjoys coordinating the Midwifery Group Practice she is working in, but that she has no formal managerial or leadership training. She feels this may be negatively impacting her effectiveness in her role.

Gail (see Example 7.2 overleaf) works in isolation in a role that relies on her ability to have knowledge of and apply the most current clinical knowledge and skills in her practice in as timely a manner as possible. She

EXAMPLE 7.1: Continuing professional development (CPD) for a midwife manager of a metropolitan-hospital-based Midwifery Group Practice (MGP)

Identified learning need	Learning plan	Activity undertaken	Reflection on activity	Relevance to NMBA Midwife standards for practice (2018)	CPD hours
I started managing my MGP in late 2015 but I don't have any management training. I think I could be more effective as a manager if I knew more about management theory and practice.	I plan to identify an experienced manager in my organisation and ask them to mentor me. I also plan to enrol in the Health Department's 'Management for Midwives' 12-week day release course.	21 January: I approached Margaret on Ward 4 and asked her to mentor me – she was delighted and agreed immediately. We meet next month for the first time. I also put in my application for the 'Midwives' Management' course after talking to my own manager and getting her support. 13 February: Met with Margaret for an hour and together we put together a learning plan for me. We agreed to meet monthly.	13 February: This first mentoring meeting was excellent, but I forgot to take a notebook! I will definitely take one next time – or I might even ask Margaret if she minds me recording the conversation because she's so full of useful information, I would like to be able to listen again to the conversation.	2. The midwife will … engage in professional relationships with other health practitioners 2.7. develops, maintains and concludes professional relationships in a way that differentiates the boundaries between professional and personal relationships 6.1. actively contributes to quality improvement … activities 6.4. provides … effective and timely direction, allocation, delegation, teaching and supervision	0.5 1.0

EXAMPLE 7.2: CPD for a midwife working in a remote community

Identified learning need	Learning plan	Activity undertaken	Reflection on activity	Relevance to NMBA Midwife standards for practice (2018)	CPD hours
I work in an isolated setting and I don't get to discuss latest best evidence with other health professionals very often. This means the care I give probably isn't always best available evidence based.	I will join the remote area health professionals' practice development network and attend the monthly meetings by videoconference.	29 February: I contacted the Chair of the remote area health professionals' practice development network and requested to join. The email I received back was very welcoming. The first meeting is in two weeks. 14 March: Joined my first remote area health professionals' practice development network where three new research papers were discussed that are relevant to my practice.	14 March: This is going to be so useful! I was invited to say what sort of practice areas I'm interested in so the group can include an item relevant to it at each meeting. I was also asked to find a piece of research and present it in three meetings' time!	1. The midwife supports women's wellbeing by providing safe, quality midwifery healthcare using the best available evidence and resources, with the principles of primary healthcare and cultural safety as foundations for practice 1.2. accesses, analyses, and uses the best available evidence, that includes research findings, for safe, quality midwifery practice 6.1. actively contributes to quality improvement and research activities	0.5 2.0

recognises that her ability to do this would be improved if she were part of a professional network of people in the same area of care as herself who could share the latest best evidence with her.

It is clear from these two examples that every registered midwife's continuing professional development action plan is going to be very different.

Once learning needs have been identified, the midwife can then plan how best to attain them. The continuing professional development plan is simply the list of activities the midwife will undertake, or the resources they will access, to enable or improve their capacity to perform their role. In Jenny's case (Example 7.1), she could plan to establish and maintain a formal mentorship arrangement with a more experienced colleague through which she could develop her managerial expertise; she might also plan to enrol in a management skills workshop or a course of study. Gail (Example 7.2) might choose to find and join a network of similar colleagues who share information regularly, or join and become active in a relevant professional organisation.

Evaluating continuing professional development activities

The purpose of this phase of the continuing professional development cycle is for the individual to determine how the new knowledge and/or skills attained through the identified learning and development activities have been applied to their own practice. If we revisit Jenny (Example 7.1), she might provide a reflective journal from her mentoring sessions or her formal learning wherein she describes how she applies what she is learning to her role and what, if any, subsequent improvements she sees as a result. In Gail's case (Example 7.2), she might keep notes of discussions she has with her new network about the latest developments in her field and document, through reflective journalling, how she is translating the new evidence she is learning about into practice.

True to the cyclical nature of the continuing professional development process, this phase helps reveal additional knowledge and skill learning needs that will inform the next continuing professional development

EXAMPLE 7.3: CPD for a midwife working in a university as a midwifery lecturer

Identified learning need	Learning plan	Activity undertaken	Date	Reflection on activity	CPD hours
I need to ensure that how I teach reflects the latest best evidence in terms of effective educational techniques for blended learning.	Subscribe to the quarterly *Journal of Fantastic Midwifery Teaching*'s contents list alerts, and select one relevant article in each issue to read and reflect on in terms of how I can apply the recommendations to my teaching practice.	Subscribed to the quarterly *Journal of Fantastic Midwifery Teaching*'s new issue contents alerts. Read January issue contents list and selected appropriate article: 'Creating engaging online discussion forums to optimise learning'. Read April issue contents list and selected appropriate article: 'Designing effective student peer teaching and learning activities'.	January January April	This article gave me some great ideas that have been shown to be effective through research about how to get students using, and learning from, online discussion forums. I can use these ideas in the learning platform at university. Although I have included peer assessment in my teaching previously, I haven't tried peer teaching before; this article provided me with information on how to apply this approach. I will introduce it into one of the obstetric emergency workshops next semester with close supervision by an experienced facilitator and evaluate students' outcomes and opinions of it.	0.5 1.5 1.5

plan. Referring again to our two midwives, Jenny might realise that in addition to developing her managerial capabilities, she also needs to further develop her leadership skills, and Gail might realise that she needs to become more proficient in critically analysing and discussing research papers relevant to her practice area to be able to decide what evidence is useful to apply.

A further example of one aspect of a continuing professional development plan that relates to the practice of a midwife in a non-clinical role is provided in Example 7.3.

Communicating Competence for Registered Nurse Practice

Lisa Devey

Nursing careers provide opportunities to work in many different areas of nursing and to take on a variety of roles. The following discussion relates to a particular role as a registered nurse in a general practice. This organisation had recently procured a number of primary care practices, in both rural and urban settings. The practices were streamlined to operate as a collective, bringing together a workforce that had previously been managing independently. The circumstances of this role made apparent, early in this transition, the need to be very clear about registered nurse accountabilities. The work setting was not like a tertiary hospital with extensive and detailed organisational policies and procedures, and with more senior or experienced registered nurses who might provide clarification or support as needed. As the only registered nurse in the setting, there was accountability, both directly and indirectly, for the enrolled nurses who were employed across the four practices.

An important step was writing a professional development plan to better understand this new role. Accessing and reading the National Practice Standards for Nurses in General Practice and the associated toolkit (Australian Nursing and Midwifery Federation 2005, 2014), in conjunction with the position description, helped to identify knowledge and skill gaps and to inform a structured plan designed to address these gaps. This process was also a prompt to check the NMBA standards for the registered nurse. Fortunately, the general practice standards aligned easily with the NMBA registered nurse standards that were in use at that time, so the competency and learning plan mapped easily to both standards. This process allowed for greater confidence in understanding the registered nurse's responsibilities for supervising the enrolled nursing practice and enabled clear discussion with work colleagues about how to manage the registered nurse accountability for enrolled nurses' practice in geographically diverse settings.

An unanticipated outcome from developing the learning plan was that it made more obvious the existing knowledge, skills and attributes that were relevant to the general practice context. In particular, skill sets around health promotion and the management of systems were readily transferable to this new setting. These skills related to the national health reforms, including chronic disease prevention and aged care. It was the registered nurse's responsibility to ensure that any implemented changes not only improved efficiencies within the practice but also were patient-focused and linked to outcomes. Using a structured approach, and regular reflection and evaluation of the professional development plan, helped in identifying ways to measure outcomes that also showed the development of new knowledge and skills, as well as to demonstrate the contribution to colleagues and the overall work of the general practice.

See Examples 7.4 and 7.5 for examples of professional development plans for clinical and non-clinical roles for nurses in general practice. Please remember CPD hours should be included as in Example 7.3.

How to evaluate your professional development plan

One of the fundamental aspects of developing a professional development plan is the ability to evaluate and reflect on the plan. The smaller workforce in the general practice setting can lead to professional or geographical isolation, and such settings may often lack a leadership structure, making it more challenging to talk through ideas with professional colleagues or managers.

Text continues on p. 99

EXAMPLE 7.4: A professional development learning plan for the clinical registered nurse in a general practice setting

Date	Areas I have identified that I need to further develop	*Maps to the registered nurse standards for practice (2016)	Professional development activity/plan	Evaluation/reflection
Self-assessment January Review March	I need to know more about general practice standards, guidelines, regulations and legislation specifically.	1.4: Complies with legislation, common law, policies, guidelines and other standards or requirements relevant to the context of practice when making decisions. 2.9: Reports notifiable conduct of health professionals, health workers and others.	Review all relevant state/territory legislation relevant to nursing practice. Familiarise myself with direct and indirect supervision guidelines. Familiarise myself with the NMBA registration standards and the decision-making framework. Read up about immunisation policy and procedures. Attend upcoming immunisation training.	Am now able to identify where to access relevant state legislation. SA Health was a useful resource for this, as well as the RACGP guidelines and the immunisation handbook. Researching immunisation policy and attending a training update helped me to identify that we were not accurately recording the temperature of the fridge. I identified a gap with checking emergency equipment in the practice. I have now implemented a whiteboard system so all staff can easily identify when the immunisation fridge, emergency trolley, drug cupboard and stock are checked in line with policy.
Self-assessment January Review March	I want to actively build and maintain professional relationships with other nurses and regularly engage in professional development activities.	2.7: Actively fosters a culture of safety and learning that includes engaging with health professionals and others, to share knowledge and practice that supports person-centred care. 3.3: Uses a lifelong learning approach for continuing professional development of self and others.	Identify a mentor (nurse in general practice) outside of the organisation. Join any relevant professional groups. Develop my own personal continuing professional development calendar, and identify relevant professional development opportunities throughout the year.	Through a pharmaceutical representative, I was introduced to a chronic disease nurse. Have since been working with my mentor to develop strategies to streamline care planning and assessments. Have joined the Australian Practice Nurse Association and will be attending their conference for national networking opportunities and to hear professional updates. I have arranged regular nursing meetings with nurses across all the sites to share information and knowledge. Meeting minutes allow us to track any actions. I have my own continuing professional development calendar as a spreadsheet and have distributed such calendars to all the nurses across the practices. I have identified some useful resources through this process.

Continued

EXAMPLE 7.4: A professional development learning plan for the clinical registered nurse in a general practice setting—cont'd

Date	Areas I have identified that I need to further develop	*Maps to the registered nurse standards for practice (2016)	Professional development activity/plan	Evaluation/reflection
Self-assessment January Review March	I want to explore further how to effectively implement evidence-based health promotion and preventative care relevant to the practice community.	6: Provides safe, appropriate and responsive quality nursing practice. 7: Evaluates outcomes to inform nursing practice.	Attend upcoming training on chronic disease management in general practice. I would like to develop a care plan/assessment system that actually measures patient outcomes.	Through searching for chronic disease management sessions and general practice/primary healthcare colleagues, I identified a chronic disease nurse who develops measurable care plans and I used this to streamline all care plans and assessments across practices so that all nurses are using the same template. This will assist with reporting consistency and review processes. I have now linked some of the chronic disease plans to risk assessments. This will help patients see how changes they are making are positively impacting on their health and assist them in taking control over their illness. Plan to do training in motivational interviewing to assist me to work with patients and have arranged to spend a day with a registered nurse I met at the APNA conference to see how they approach care plans and assessment in their practice.
Self-assessment January Review March	To demonstrate greater proficiency in the use of information technology, clinical software and decision support tools to underpin healthcare delivery.	4: Comprehensively conducts assessments.	I would like to learn how to use the medical software more efficiently in my practice to help identify potential consumers and link them in to healthcare opportunities. Training booked with Divisions of General Practice – how to use Pencat and interrogate the clinical software.	Since undertaking the training, I have been working with reception staff and nursing staff to refine our recall system. We have now improved our systems and increased the billings of incentive payments that were previously being missed. I have also worked with the GPs in streamlining their referral letters across the practices to ensure the new branding is correct and there is no confusion for patients.

Note: *These competency standards have now been replaced with practice standards for the registered nurse (NMBA).

EXAMPLE 7.5: A professional development learning plan for the non-clinical registered nurse in a general practice setting

Date	Areas I have identified that I need to further develop	*Maps to the national competency standards for the registered nurse	Professional development activity/plan	Evaluation/Reflection
Self-assessment January Review March	Advocates for the role of nursing in general practice.	3.6: Actively engages with the profession.	Seek opportunities to promote nursing in general practice and the role of the nurse in general practice. Share with and impart knowledge to nursing colleagues and the profession.	I have assisted the ANMF (Federal Office) in running focus groups for the review of the National Practice Standards for Nurses in General Practice. These focus groups will enable nurses in general practice to inform the revision of the standards and participate in a national research project. I have linked in with local universities to run sessions on nursing in general practice as a career pathway. Taking on my new role as a liaison officer, I have been able to facilitate nursing students in undertaking placements in general practice. This role enables me to advocate for nursing in general practice at an undergraduate level and encourage students to consider this as a career pathway for succession planning.
Self-assessment January Review March	Demonstrates nursing leadership.	2.8: participates in and/ or leads collaborative practice.	Link in with professional working groups. Seek out mentoring and leadership training to assist in my role as liaison officer and support person for nurses in general practice.	I have identified and joined a Primary Health Care Nurses Mentor Panel. The panel allows me to meet with experts in the field and share knowledge to bring back to my network of nurses. Have also enrolled in Primary Health Care Nursing Leadership and Mentoring Training to further develop my skills in providing collegial support.

Continued

EXAMPLE 7.5: A professional development learning plan for the non-clinical registered nurse in a general practice setting—cont'd

Date	Areas I have identified that I need to further develop	*Maps to the national competency standards for the registered nurse	Professional development activity/plan	Evaluation/Reflection
Self-assessment January Review March	Contributes to quality improvement and research activities to monitor and improve the standard of care provided in general practice.	1.7: contributes to quality improvement and relevant research.	I would like to learn how to access and implement evidence-based practice standards/guidelines into general practice so that I can impart this knowledge to my colleagues. I have identified a Best Practice Spotlight Learning Institute (BPSO) at the ANMF (SA Branch) to learn how to implement evidence-based practice in the workplace.	This learning institute helped me to identify and access evidence-based tools to implement in the primary healthcare setting. I was also able to network with other primary healthcare nurses at the institute and have been given a folder of templates to assist in developing policies and procedures. I have used these templates as a guide for new nurses in general practice to help implement policies and procedures when they start at a practice. I have arranged a speaker to run a professional development session with the nurses who form part of the network I work with, to understand the importance of underpinning their practice in evidence and evaluating practice. This will have an overall positive impact on outcomes for patients.

Note: *These competency standards have now been replaced with practice standards for the registered nurse (NMBA).

As identified in the National Practice Standards for Nurses in General Practice, a nurse's performance can be separated into two distinct areas: clinical and organisational (Australian Nursing and Midwifery Federation 2014). The Australian Nursing and Midwifery Federation (2014) identified the need for professional and clinical understanding for the peer review/evaluation process. Professional organisations such as the Australian Nursing and Midwifery Federation and the Australian Primary Health Care Nurses Association have developed templates and tools to assist in this process of evaluation.

Communicating Competence for Enrolled Nurse Practice

Síobhán Bidgood

The professional development requirements of enrolled nurses are similar to, yet distinct from, those of registered nurses and midwives. The NMBA Enrolled Nurse Standards for Practice (Nursing and Midwifery Board of Australia 2016b) provide a benchmark for competency and a means to measure the individual enrolled nurses' needs in maintaining their competence.

The previous chapters of this book describe how to produce a portfolio to enhance and evidence professional competence and ongoing practice development. They incorporate how to assess your professional development needs and maintain an evidence trail of the implementation and evaluation of your development plan. As with any health professional, a useful tool for the enrolled nurse is the annual performance review meeting, which provides an opportunity to review and document a performance plan, ideally in a collaborative meeting format. In addition to a meeting of this nature providing an important basis for developing a continuing professional development plan, the very nature of the collaboration is a demonstration of the enrolled nurse adhering to their practice standard of working with and under the supervision of a registered nurse.

The NMBA Enrolled Nurse Standards for Practice outline three domains of practice, namely:

- professional and collaborative practice
- provision of care
- reflective and analytical practice (Nursing and Midwifery Board of Australia 2016b, p. 2).

It is useful to consider examples that relate to the domains of the enrolled nurse standards for practice, as a way of putting these standards into practice (see Table 7.1). Please remember CPD hours should be included as in Example 7.3.

TABLE 7.1
Communicating competence for enrolled nurse practice

Date	Identified learning need	Domain and standard	Action plan	Reflection on activity specific to practice
February	Need to know more about social media in relation to upholding a person's rights, confidentiality, dignity and respect.	Domain: Professional and Collaborative Practice. Standard: 2	Access the social media guidelines published on the NMBA website. Access and read workplace social media policy. Complete the unit related to social media in the mandatory training packages. Discuss issues with senior colleagues.	Learned the maintenance of client and colleague privacy is an important consideration with the use of social media posing special challenges in terms of maintaining both privacy and confidentiality. For example: inappropriate use of Facebook and Snapchat to post photos or information about staff or clients.

TABLE 7.1

Communicating competence for enrolled nurse practice—cont'd

Date	Identified learning need	Domain and standard	Action plan	Reflection on activity specific to practice
February	I am working with clients in the Neurostimulation Department. Have an understanding of basic assessment but need to know more about specific neurostimulation assessment techniques for this client group.	Domain: Provision of Care. Standard: 4	Complete training in neurostimulation nursing.	Completed the training course and learned more about both ECT and TMS.

Communicating Competence for Practice in Occupational Therapy

Susan Gilbert-Hunt

To maintain registration, occupational therapists are required to provide evidence of developing and extending knowledge, skills and competence in relation to practice standards. Like all registered health practitioners, all registered occupational therapists are required to undertake a minimum number of hours of continuing professional development on an annual basis (Occupational Therapy Board of Australia 2012). This requirement is currently set at 30 hours and is to be made up of a mixture of activities, as outlined in Table 7.2.

At the point of registration renewal, occupational therapists are required to make a declaration of compliance and to keep and retain detailed records of all activities for a period of five years. The Occupational Therapy Board of Australia undertakes random periodic audits that require the practitioner to produce, within one month of the audit notice, their continuing professional development record and portfolio of evidence for the identified year.

Planning your continuing professional development

A structure and process for undertaking continuing professional development needs careful planning, monitoring and evaluation. First of all, set two to three goals with clear, measurable outcomes that can be evidenced. To develop an effective plan, it is necessary to determine where you are currently positioned in relation to your practice and what you need to focus on over the 12 months. It may be helpful to review the previous continuing professional development plan and outcomes to determine the extent to which objectives were met, and to take note of strategies that worked well

and those that were not as effective. As well as looking back, also look forward to where you want to be in the next 12 months and consider potential learning and development opportunities.

Below are two examples of planning for continuing professional development.

Example: Jan

Jan graduated five years ago and worked in a range of organisations that focused mainly on adult rehabilitation services in hospitals and community settings. She recently moved to a large rural town and secured a position on the Children's Unit, which next year will include being part of the paediatric outreach team. She will be providing services to families in rural and remote areas and working within Indigenous communities one day a week. Jan sets her goals and outcomes for the next 12 months and also has ideas of how she will achieve them using formal and informal learning activities to comply with the continuing professional development categories of the Board (see Example 7.6). While opportunities for these will arise from time to time, it is important to have some activities planned in advance to ensure that learning goals are met.

Example: Matt

Matt is a newly graduated occupational therapist and has just started his first job with an aged care provider. He feels there is a lot he doesn't know and wants to ensure he uses the continuing professional development process to support his transition to practice. On his clinical placements, he always received positive feedback about his interpersonal skills and ability to connect with

TABLE 7.2

Occupational therapy CPD categories

Formal learning activities	Informal learning activities	Engagement with profession
Maximum of 25 hours of CPD per year	**Maximum of 25 hours of CPD per year**	**Maximum of 10 hours of CPD per year**
Examples:	Examples:	Examples:
• completing tertiary study • completing training course • completing work-based learning that involved assessed activity • attendance at conference, workshop, seminar • undertaking research and presentation of work (must be substantive, reference- and evidence-based) • publishing in a peer-reviewed journal • authoring a book chapter • attending journal club • developing evidence-based practice resources (e.g. systematic review) • distance/online learning that includes an assessment or certificate evidencing learning outcomes.	• private study such as reading books or journals • completing case reviews/ presentations with colleagues • examining and reflecting on evidence-based resources and translating them into practice • participating in a community of practice, with a record of activities completed • reflective journalling, which must be detailed and focus on developing competence and quality practice • online learning through chat rooms, list-serves, etc. • receiving supervision or mentoring from an occupational therapist (record of the supervision, discussion involved and documentation of outcomes).	• completing accreditation activities (inspection teams, evaluation of accreditation reports) • participating in activities to improve practice or minimise risk that involve evaluation and reporting • participating in a clinical audit or similar review activity • supervising undergraduate or postgraduate occupational therapy students • supervising occupational therapists undertaking a practice audit or program of supervised practice • providing supervision or mentoring of an occupational therapist (record of the supervision, discussion involved and documentation of outcomes) • participating in interest groups, committees, boards, etc., with a focus on health or professional issues • presenting in-service or training to health professionals or carers.

and respond to clients. He also feels relatively confident about the occupational therapy process. However, he received consistent feedback that he needed to further improve his information-gathering and report-writing skills. With this in mind, he develops the continuing professional development plan outlined in Example 7.7.

Having made a detailed plan for continuing professional development, it is also necessary to keep a log of activities and to evaluate your progress. You can use any format you prefer. The case example given here is based on the template provided by the Occupational Therapy Board of Australia. In addition to the log, you must keep all your evidence of these activities. This documentation needs to include the time spent in formal and informal learning activities, as well as on engagement with the profession. Goals and outcomes are important to describe, as per Example 7.8.

EXAMPLE 7.6: Jan's goals and outcomes

Goal	Outcome	Potential activities	Evidence
Improve knowledge and skill in providing culturally safe and responsive care.	Increased confidence in providing therapy services to children and families who come from culturally and linguistically diverse backgrounds.	1 Set up meetings with mentor via OT Australia and a local person (informal). 2 Undertake cultural training workshop run by rural department of health (formal). 3 Read journal articles on culturally safe practice (informal). 4 Maintain a reflective journal with a focus on culturally responsive practice and skills (informal). 5 Have mentor or supervisor provide feedback on session with family.	1 Record of meetings, discussions and outcomes. 2 Attendance/assessment certificate. 3 Documentation of journal articles read and implications for practice. 4 Document journal writing sessions with regular précis of themes and implications for practice. 5 Notes from mentor/supervisor feedback.
Improve knowledge of living conditions and likely health issues prevalent in children living in rural and remote areas.	Able to respond to the health needs of children and families in rural and remote communities.	1 Discuss with mentor prevalent health issues and OT practice in rural areas (informal). 2 Participate in the OT4OT rural and remote online group (informal). 3 Research health conditions in children living in rural and remote Australia (informal).	1 Record of meetings, discussions and outcomes. 2 Record of participation and notes on practice implications (screenshots, if appropriate). 3 Record of database searches, articles read and notes on practice implications.

EXAMPLE 7.7: Matt's continuing professional development plan

Goal	Outcome	Potential activities	Evidence
Develop knowledge of the aged care system and practice.	Competent in providing a range of OT services to older clients, including those with dementia.	1 Attend organisation's orientation workshop (formal). 2 Identify a suitable OT supervisor (informal). 3 Review university notes and resources (informal). 4 Join OT aged care interest groups (engagement with profession). 5 Undertake Understanding Dementia MOOC with university (formal). 6 Maintain a reflective journal that focuses on practice knowledge and skills in aged care.	1 Attendance certificate. 2 Record of meetings, discussions and outcomes. 3 Record of time spent reviewing, with notes on implications for practice. 4 Record of attendance, notes and reflection of practice implications. 5 Completion certificate. 6 Document journal writing sessions with regular précis of themes and implications for practice.
Develop documentation and report-writing skills.	Competent and efficient in documentation skills.	1 Review documentation standards within the organisation and develop personalised checklist (informal). 2 Have supervisor regularly review documentation and provide feedback.	1 Checklist. 2 Record of supervisor meetings and feedback on documentation.
Improve skills in assessing clients' accommodation needs.	Confident to complete assessment and make recommendation about accommodation needs.	1 Review assessment procedures with supervisor. 2 Review relevant journal articles. 3 Supervisor to review performance of assessment.	1 Record of meetings and implications for practice. 2 Documentation of journals read and implications for practice. 3 Record of activity and feedback.

EXAMPLE 7.8: Goals and objectives in an occupational therapist's CPD plan

Goals	Outcomes
Improve knowledge and skill in providing culturally safe and responsive care.	Increased confidence in providing therapy services to children and families who come from culturally and linguistically diverse backgrounds.
Improve knowledge of living conditions and likely health issues prevalent in children living in rural and remote areas.	Able to respond to the health needs of children and families in rural and remote communities.

Communicating Competence for Practice in Paramedicine

Joe Acker

Paramedics in Australia and New Zealand

Paramedicine became the fifteenth nationally regulated health profession in Australia under the Health Practitioner Regulation National Law Act (National Law) on 1 December 2018 (Paramedicine Board of Australia 2018a). It is anticipated that paramedics in New Zealand will also be regulated under the *Health Practitioners Competence Assurance (HPCA) Act 2003* in the not-too-distant future (Paramedics Australasia 2016). The recognition of paramedicine as a health profession can be partially attributed to major advancements in paramedic education that transitioned from on-the-job training provided by state and territory ambulance services to vocational qualifications and, more recently, university tertiary education with undergraduate qualifications required for entry to practice (Brooks et al. 2018, O'Meara et al. 2017, Tolari & Acker 2013).

The Paramedicine Board of Australia established a comprehensive description of the professional capabilities for registered paramedics in 2018. These capabilities identify the knowledge, skills and professional attributes needed for safe and competent practice of paramedicine in Australia and draw on the *Professional Competency Standards – Paramedics Version 2.2* 2013 published by the Council of Ambulance Authorities and the *Australasian Competency Standards for Paramedics 2011* published by Paramedicine Australasia. The paramedic capabilities are divided into five domains including: professional and ethical conduct; professional communications and collaboration; evidence-based practice and professional learning; safety risk management and quality assurance; and paramedicine practice (Paramedicine Board of Australia 2019). Paramedics are expected to maintain, update and advance these capabilities throughout their careers, which requires ongoing continuing professional development (CPD).

Planning and recording your paramedic professional development

With paramedics now registered with the Paramedicine Board of Australia under the Australian Health Practitioner Regulation Agency there is a mandatory requirement to participate in and keep an accurate record of at least 30 hours of annual continuing professional development activities with a minimum of eight hours of interactive CPD with other practitioners. These requirements will apply not only to those in clinical practice but also to those paramedics working in non-clinical paramedic roles including administration, research, management, advisory, regulation or education. All paramedics should take personal ownership for their professional development; no longer can they rely on their employer to provide all the training required (Gent 2016). This means that paramedics must move beyond employer-provided training that requires no independent thought to an educational approach of self-directed learning that will require an attitude change across the whole profession. This *cultural revolution* starts with you becoming a champion for professional development across the profession by creating a personal portfolio and professional development plan and then encouraging your paramedic classmates, colleagues, preceptors, mentors, supervisors and educators to do the same.

A structured approach to continuing professional development

Every paramedic is responsible for their own professional development, and the activities in your learning plan should fill learning gaps that are specific to your role and to the work environment. The professional development plan should be useful and relevant to 'lifelong learning', help you to advance in your organisation, and be within an approved structure that meets the standards set by the regulator. Suggested steps in the development of a learning plan are as follows:

1 Use reflective techniques to identify areas of practice that need to be enhanced and what is to be achieved in areas of deficiency (e.g. theoretical understanding, skills competence, soft skills).
2 Develop SMART learning outcomes (specific, measurable, attainable, results-focused, time-focused).
3 Select a suitable learning activity to achieve each learning outcome while matching this to personal learning preferences. (See Table 7.3 for examples of paramedic learning activities.)
4 Use reflective and reflexive techniques to evaluate the learning activity and the learning experience to review how it helped achieve the identified learning outcomes.
5 Use your portfolio to record areas for development, learning outcomes, learning activities and reflections about competence development after completing the learning activity (Martin 2006).

Many different things can motivate the self-identification of learning needs. For example, you may be reading a new clinical protocol and find that you haven't kept up to date with some of the latest pharmacology; or maybe, when reviewing a list of competencies that your paramedic student is expected to perform, you recognise that you haven't performed some of these skills in the last year or more. Regardless of the motivation, you need to dedicate time and effort to critically and constructively assessing your own practice to identify weaknesses and learning gaps.

After determining your learning gaps, the next step is to identify key specific learning outcomes to address these gaps. Learning outcomes help you to focus your learning on specific areas that allow you to use your time most efficiently. Using the example above, by recognising a weakness in your knowledge of the new pharmacology – ketamine, for example – you could develop a few simple learning outcomes, such as:

1 Describe the classification, indications, contraindications, actions, complications, doses and routes for the administration of ketamine before my next set of shifts.

2 Calculate the correct adult and paediatric doses of ketamine for a range of patient weights before my next set of shifts.

These two learning outcomes are SMART – that is, they are specific (you know what you need to do), measurable (you know when you achieve them), attainable (they are not difficult to achieve), results-focused (you need to know your pharmacology in your job as a paramedic) and time-focused (you have set a deadline to achieve these outcomes before your next set of shifts).

Once you have identified your learning gap, and developed some SMART learning outcomes, you need to find appropriate learning activities that will help you to achieve your learning outcomes. Remember that learning activities don't need to be formal education or training courses. They can be informal and self-directed activities; however, evidence suggests that interactive and interprofessional education activities facilitate effective learning (Paramedicine Board of Australia 2018b). A list of potential paramedic learning activities is provided in Table 7.3. For our example of learning about a new medication such as ketamine, there are a number of possible learning activities available to you:

- Complete an e-learning package provided by your ambulance service or your professional association that deals specifically with ketamine. Both national paramedic associations, Paramedics Australasia (www.paramedics.org) and the Australian and New Zealand College of Paramedicine (www.anzcp.org.au), offer e-learning courses to members and both provide online portfolios for members to track their CPD, include personal reflections, and report on their CPD if audited.
- Go to a bookstore, a public library or your local university and find texts on pharmacology. Read what you find most relevant and complete the assessment activities usually included in such resources.
- Make an appointment with one of the paramedic clinical educators at your ambulance station or a paramedic mentor to discuss the use of ketamine in the paramedic practice setting.
- Attend a conference or workshop where an expert guest speaker presents new research or case reports of the use of ketamine in paramedic practice.

TABLE 7.3

Examples of paramedic learning activities

The Paramedicine Board of Australia requires a minimum of 30 hours of continuing professional development per year with at least eight hours of interactive or interprofessional learning with other practitioners.

WORK-BASED LEARNING
- Mentor students or new staff and assist them in developing learning plans.
- Share information from sources or workshops with colleagues.
- Reflect on a patient experience that could have gone better and investigate the literature or discuss the case with a trusted peer for ways to improve your practice.
- Participate in a clinical audit or clinical review of patient healthcare records.
- Start or participate in journal clubs at work and post interesting articles.
- Take an acting role in a different part of your organisation and document your observations and reflections of working in this role.

PROFESSIONAL ACTIVITIES
- Become a member in a professional peak body such as Paramedics Australasia or the Australian and New Zealand College of Paramedicine.
- Volunteer as a committee or board member for a peak body, council or regulator.
- Be an examiner, accreditor or auditor for the professional council or regulatory body.
- Shadow a senior nurse or doctor in the emergency department.
- Do a 'ride-along' with an ambulance service overseas and develop an international network to share best practices.
- Deliver a guest lecture or tutorial at a university paramedic course or professional development event.
- Present at a paramedicine- or medicine-related conference.
- Organise and facilitate a formal journal club.
- Supervise research.
- Be an expert witness.

FORMAL EDUCATION AND TRAINING
- Attend an ambulance service training course.
- Complete a medical certification course such as Advanced Cardiac Life Support or Paediatric Advanced Life Support.
- Enrol in a postgraduate course such as a Graduate Diploma in Intensive Care Paramedicine or a Master's Degree by research.
- Attend a conference.
- Write articles or papers.
- Teach or lecture paramedicine students.

TABLE 7.3

Examples of paramedic learning activities—cont'd

SELF-DIRECTED LEARNING
- Engage in FOAMed (Free Open Access Medical education) by following quality websites and making valuable social media contacts.
- Complete online e-learning packages.
- Read journal articles.
- Keep a record or file of your learning journey.

OTHER
- Teach a CPR course to local groups.
- Attend schools or public events to demonstrate the role of the ambulance service (i.e. when to call 000 [in Australia, or 112 on a mobile phone; in New Zealand, the emergency number is 111]).
- Participate in relevant volunteer work.

Source: Adapted from Health and Care Professions Council 2014.

- Review Free Open Access Medical education (FOAMed) (Johnston & Acker 2015, Nickson & Cadogan 2014) and find learning resources on social media (Twitter, LinkedIn, Facebook) or from online blogs and YouTube videos that address your learning outcomes. For example, you may use the free site Prehospital and Retrieval Medicine (PHARM), which has a range of podcasts, articles and learning tools for paramedics and emergency physicians (Prehospital and Retrieval Medicine 2015).

During and after the learning activities, take time to evaluate and consider the value of the learning experience. Everyone has a preferred learning style. Ask yourself questions such as: Did the learning activity work for you? If it did, document it in your portfolio so that you can return to these types of activities in the future. If the learning activity wasn't effective, why not? What can you do differently next time to make it more valuable? Remember that the Board requires you to collect evidence for a range of different learning activities. Chapter 3 in this book discussed the importance of reflection and reflective practice, and by now you may understand the links between being reflexive and reflective when taking responsibility for your own learning. Reflexivity should not be confused with reflectivity. *Reflection* is an important tool for learning that happens *after* an activity is complete, where we identify what we learnt and how we can do it differently next time. *Reflexivity*, on the other hand, is the practice of engaging *in the moment*, to understand your thoughts and feelings of a learning experience while still engaging in that experience. Reflective and reflexive observations should be recorded in your professional portfolio, as these are very important artefacts that help you to become a reflective practitioner.

The final step in a structured professional development plan is to collect everything in your portfolio and document a final self-evaluation of your learning journey over a set period of time with a new plan for the future. Regardless of whether your portfolio is paper-based or electronic, casual or complex, you should record a description of the learning gap you identified, a list of your SMART learning outcomes, evidence of the learning activities you completed, reflections on the value of the learning activities, and the final reflective evaluation of this educational experience. The Paramedicine Board of Australia requires that the CPD portfolio be retained for at least five years because these records may be required for a CPD audit or if required by the Board as part of an investigation into a complaint (Paramedicine Board of Australia 2018b).

This structured approach to professional development for paramedics is relatively straightforward and flexible enough to work for a wide range of individuals and, indeed, for many different health professions. Another activity that can be used to assess and record your professional development is through the use of a competency profile.

Communicating Competence for Practice in Pharmacy

Kearney Gleadhill

The Pharmacy Board of Australia (PharmBA), as part of its registration standards and guidelines, has developed a standard for continuing professional development (Pharmacy Board of Australia 2015a). This standard and the associated guidelines apply to applicants for general registration and all registered pharmacists, including those changing registration type. They do not apply to pharmacists with non-practising registration, or to students. All activities that a pharmacist counts towards their annual continuing professional development requirements must be relevant to their intended or current scope of practice. The PharmBA website provides details of the relevant requirements for registered pharmacists in Australia.

The continuing professional development requirements are the same for pharmacists working part-time and full-time, and address instances such as where a pharmacist has a leave of absence from the profession. Before applying for general registration, or renewal of general registration, the Recency of Practice Registration Standard for pharmacists (Pharmacy Board of Australia 2015b) requires the pharmacist to have practised for a minimum of:

- 450 hours in the preceding three-year period, or
- 150 hours in the preceding 12-month period.

This practice can have occurred in either Australia or New Zealand, with other countries being considered by the PharmBA on a case-by-case basis. Records of practice undertaken during the previous three full registration periods should be maintained.

Planning your continuing professional development

The PharmBA guidelines on continuing professional development (2015a) state that pharmacists should ensure that they meet all of the Board's continuing professional development standards by:

- developing and maintaining their continuing professional development plan
- selecting appropriate activities to address the competencies identified in the continuing professional development plan which are relevant to their scope of practice
- maintaining detailed records of activities undertaken
- ensuring that these records can be verified.

The PharmBA standards and guidelines can be used by pharmacists to assist with the identification of their scope of practice, determination of their professional development needs, and the creation of a personalised professional practice profile. This profile can be used to identify the competency standards relevant to the role performed by individual pharmacists (i.e. their scope of practice) and, subsequently, any areas to target for continuing professional development activities. Self-reflection and performance appraisal can also be used to assist in identification of learning needs.

There are three types of continuing professional development activity groups: Groups 1, 2 and 3. They are defined by the PharmBA as shown in Table 7.4.

Of the eight domains of professional responsibility in the National Competency Standards Framework for Pharmacists in Australia (Pharmacy Board of Australia 2014), the first two have been deemed universally applicable and should be included in the continuing professional development plan. The presence or absence of domains three to eight may vary significantly in the professional practice profiles of individual pharmacists.

'Scope of practice' for pharmacists refers to the professional role and services that a pharmacist has

TABLE 7.4

Continuing professional development activity groups

Activity type	Description (from PharmBA guidelines on CPD)	CPD credit per hour of activity	Examples
Information accessed without assessment	Didactic presentations, and activities with little or no attendee interaction.	1	Watching/listening to presentations; reading journals; preparing for external review; researching a topic to support individual patient care.
Knowledge or skills improved with assessment	Activities where the participant's acquisition of knowledge or skills can be demonstrated – for example, through successful completion of some form of assessment.	2	As above, but additionally includes (in relation to the CPD activity) assessment; or interaction/ discussion; or maintaining a log/ journal.
Quality or practice- improvement facilitated	Activities where an assessment of existing practice (of an individual or within a pharmacy practice), and of the needs and barriers to changes in this practice, is undertaken prior to the development of a particular activity. As a result, the activity addresses identified professional development needs with a reflection post-activity to evaluate practice change or outcomes resulting from the activity. Such an activity most likely will extend over a number of weeks or months.	3	Work undertaken for presentation of a paper/poster at a conference or publication of an article in a peer-reviewed journal; lead in workplace quality or practice improvement activities (e.g. drug utilisation review); active involvement in a special-interest group leading to demonstrated practice change; using information from a CPD activity to facilitate quality or practice improvement.

Source: Pharmacy Board of Australia 2014.

the education and competency to perform (Pharmacy Board of Australia 2015a). It is no surprise that this practice varies greatly from one pharmacist to another. Therefore, it is important to understand one's scope of practice (which can be aided by the development of a professional practice profile) so that this informs an individualised continuing professional development plan.

What continuing professional development is available for pharmacists?

Pharmacists can undertake a range of activities to meet their continuing professional development plan, such as:

- actively engaging with professional organisations
- attending relevant conferences
- reading and reflecting on journal articles
- in-house/employment-based staff development
- formal tertiary-based educational programs
- self-generated study programs.

Various resources include some that either have no cost or are available at no cost to members. The PharmBA's frequently asked questions (FAQs) document lists the following examples of organisations providing pharmacy-related continuing professional development:

- Society of Hospital Pharmacists of Australia (SHPA): www.shpa.org.au

- Pharmaceutical Society of Australia (PSA): www.psa.org.au
- Australian College of Pharmacy (ACP): www.acp.edu.au
- Pharmacy Guild of Australia (PGA): www.guild.org.au
- NPS Medicineswise: www.nps.org.au
- Medicines Safety Update: www.tga.gov.au

Many of these organisations offer relevant journals or other literature, online education, or access to conferences, workshops or seminars. It is important to remember that in-house education or training can often be included. If unsure whether an education session can be included as a part of your continuing professional development plan, review the PharmBA's *Guidelines on CPD* or *Frequently Asked Questions – CPD* publications.

For pharmacists interested in further formal educational programs, several universities offer a variety of courses or units of study.

Although PharmaBA has not specified a format for developing a continuing professional development plan, a template available on its website can assist pharmacists in doing so. The template includes the following elements:

- area identified requiring professional development (relevant competencies from competency standards framework)
- start and finish date of activity
- source of provider details
- type of activity
- topics covered during activity
- accreditation status (accredited or non-accredited)
- CPD activity group (Group 1, 2 or 3)
- how activity has impacted practice
- Pharmacy Board of Australia CPD credits.
  Key questions to be addressed in the continuing professional development plan include the following:
- What have you identified as areas that require professional development?
- What actions will you take to meet your professional development needs?

- What actions have you taken to meet your professional development needs?
- What has been the outcome of this professional development (e.g. has there been any change in practice or patient benefit)?

The pharmacist professional organisations provide members with additional resources to assist with self-assessment and continuing professional development planning, which can be useful for those who do not wish to design their own.

How to evaluate your professional development plan

As described previously, the *National Competency Standards Framework for Pharmacists in Australia* provides guidance on developing a professional practice profile. This document represents the competency standards for the entire pharmacy profession and allows individual pharmacists to determine which standards apply specifically to them. The PharmBA guidelines on continuing professional development recommend that pharmacists use this framework to determine their professional development needs. At the beginning of each continuing professional development period, a plan should be developed based on these needs, and this should be regularly reviewed and amended as additional needs evolve. For example, this would include unplanned research of an issue related to their care of an individual patient.

There are a number of ways that a pharmacist can evaluate their continuing professional development plan. Examples need to be specific to the professional group being addressed, but may include:

- outcome assessments on what has been achieved through the learning activity
- peer review opportunities to critically discuss and reflect on the learning need
- benchmarking with similar pharmacy partners.

This process must be documented as evidence of completing the cycle of continuing professional development.

Conclusion

The objective of this book has been to provide a comprehensive overview of how to develop portfolios to assist you in maintaining, enhancing and explaining your practice as a health professional. As has been detailed, portfolios can be used to develop and document your reflective analytical skills and demonstrate your learning. The capacity of individuals to undertake what is in effect a form of self-regulation of competence is inherent in the concept of a profession. As a consequence of understanding both the regulatory requirements and standards of our professions and our own abilities to meet these, we are able to self-audit and progressively remedy any shortfalls. As is evident in this text, competence is a progressive and changing entity that requires individual professionals to adjust to new information, emerging best-practice criteria and changing population needs. Importantly, by ensuring that we, as individual health professionals, are capable of making these ongoing adjustments, we contribute to the dynamic momentum of our professions in attending to emerging health priorities and population needs.

This chapter, in particular, has focused on the use of portfolios to direct and review your continuing professional development. Various health professionals have given exemplars of how they use the skills outlined in this book to attend to their ongoing registration requirements. Importantly, the respective registration Boards have specific registration requirements to be met for your individual professional group. However, in reviewing those requirements as detailed on the relevant Board website, we urge you to consider the information set out in this book, which is designed to assist you to maximise the benefits of the reflective process required. As this and earlier chapters have demonstrated, a portfolio can provide you with the opportunity to generate and update a more comprehensive range of evidence for competency to practise. Over time, this can also be used to assist you in promotion applications, registration endorsements, career planning and position applications.

References

André, K., 2010. E-portfolios for the aspiring professional. Collegian 17 (3), 119–124.

André, K., Heartfield, M., 2007. Professional Portfolios: Evidence of Competency for Nurses and Midwives. Elsevier Australia, Sydney.

Andrews, R., 2010. Argumentation in Higher Education: Improving Practice Through Theory and Research. Routledge, New York.

Asselin, M.E., Schwartz-Barcott, D., Osterman, P.A., 2012. Exploring reflection as a process embedded in experienced nurses' practice: a qualitative study. J. Adv. Nurs. 69 (4), 905–914. doi:10.1111/j.1365-2648.2012.06082.x.

Australian Commission on Safety and Quality in Health Care, 2011. Patient-centred care: improving quality and safety through partnerships with patients and consumers. ACSQHC, Sydney.

Australian Commission on Safety and Quality in Health Care, 2012. Overview of the Australian safety and quality goals for health care. 29 August. www.safetyandquality.gov.au/publications/overview-of-the-australian-safety-and-quality-goals-for-health-care. (Accessed 4 October 2019).

Australian Health Practitioner Regulation Agency, 2014. National Board policy for registered health practitioners. Social media policy. https://www.nursingmidwiferyboard.gov.au/codes-guidelines-statements/policies/social-media-policy.aspx. (Accessed 4 September 2019).

Australian Health Practitioner Regulation Agency, 2019a. Registration Standards. https://www.ahpra.gov.au/Registration/Registration-Standards.aspx. (Accessed 1 July 2019).

Australian Health Practitioner Regulation Agency, 2019b. https://www.ahpra.gov.au/. (Accessed 1 July 2019).

Australian Nursing and Midwifery Federation, 2005. Competency standards for nurses in general practice. www.anmf.org.au. (Accessed 1 October 2016).

Australian Nursing and Midwifery Federation – Federal Office, 2014. National practice standards for nurses in general practice. https://www.anmf.org.au/documents/National_Practice_Standards_for_Nurses_in_General_Practice.pdf. (Accessed 3 June 2019).

Barrett, H., 2007. Researching electronic portfolios and learner engagement: the REFLECT initiative. J. Adolesc. Adult Lit. 50 (6), 436–449.

Barrett, H., 2010. Balancing the two faces of ePortfolios. http://electronicportfolios.org/balance/index.html. (Accessed 3 June 2019).

Benner, P., Sutphen, M., Leonard, V., et al., 2010. Educating Nurses: A Call for Radical Transformation. Jossey-Bass, San Francisco, CA.

Benton, D., Perez-Raya, F., Gonzalez-Jurado, M.A., et al., 2015. Keeping pace with an ever-changing world: a policy imperative. J. Nurs. Regul. 6 (1), 20–24.

Biggs, J., Tang, C., 2011. Teaching for Quality Learning at University, fourth ed. Society for Research into Higher Education and Open University Press, McGraw-Hill, Berkshire, UK.

Bolton, G., 2005. Reflective Practice: Writing and Professional Development. Sage, London.

Branch, W.T., Paranjape, A., 2002. Feedback and reflection: teaching methods for clinical settings. Acad. Med. 77 (12), 1185–1188.

Brookhart, S.M., 2013. How to create and use rubrics for formative assessment and grading. ASCD, Alexandria, Virginia, USA.

Brooks, I.A., Grantham, H., Spencer, C., et al., 2018. A review of the literature: the transition of entry-level paramedic education in Australia from vocational to higher education (1961–2017). Australas. J. Paramed. 15 (2).

Brown, C.E., Ecoff, L., Kim, S.C., et al., 2010. Multi-institutional study of barriers to research utilisation and evidence-based practice among hospital nurses. J. Clin. Nurs. 19, 1944–1951.

Brown, D., Edwards, H., 2015. Lewis's Medical–Surgical Nursing, fourth ed. Elsevier Australia, Sydney.

Brownie, S., Bahnisch, M., Thomas, J., 2011. Exploring the literature: competency-based education and competency-based career frameworks. University of Queensland node of the Australian Health Workforce Institute in partnership with Health Workforce Australia, Adelaide.

Buckley, S., Coleman, J., Khan, K., 2010. Best evidence on the educational effects of undergraduate portfolios. Clin. Teach. 7, 187–191.

Bulman, C., 2008a. Help to get you started. In: Bulman, C., Schutz, S. (Eds.), Reflective Practice in Nursing. Blackwell, Chichester, UK, pp. 219–239, (Ch. 9).

Bulman, C., Schutz, S. (Eds.), 2008. Reflective Practice in Nursing. Blackwell, Chichester, UK.

Caldwell, L., Grobbel, C.C., 2013. The importance of reflective practice in nursing. Int. J. Caring Sci. 6 (3), 319–326.

Cashin, A., Heartfield, M., Bryce, J., et al., 2017. Standards for practice for registered nurses in Australia. Collegian 24 (3), 255–266.

Chan, W., 2014. A better norm-referenced grading using the standard deviation criteria. Teach. Learn. Med. 26 (4), 364–365.

Chertoff, J., Wright, A., Noval, M., et al., 2016. Status of portfolios in undergraduate medical education in the LCME accredited US medical school. Med. Teach. 38 (9), 886–896. doi:10.3109/0142159X.2015.1114595.

Cioffi, J.M., 2015. Insight and discovery in clinical nursing practice. Collegian 24 (2), 191–196. doi.org/10.1016/j .colegn.2015.10.004.

Clouder, L., Sellars, J., 2004. Reflective practice and clinical supervision: an interprofessional perspective. J. Adv. Nurs. 46 (3), 262–269.

Coalition of National Nursing and Midwifery Organisations, 2015. www.conno.org.au. (Accessed 27 September 2019).

College of Occupational Therapists of Nova Scotia, 2015. Continuing competency program overview. http://cotns.ca/ quality-practice/overview/. (Accessed 24 September 2019).

Colvin, E., Bacchus, R., Knight, E., et al., 2016. Exploring the way students use rubrics in the context of criterion referenced assessment. In: Davis, M., Goody, A. (Eds.), Research and Development in Higher Education: The Shape of Higher Education, vol. 39. Fremantle, Australia, pp. 42–52.

Cooper, T., Emden, C., 2001. Portfolio assessment: a guide for nurses and midwives. Praxis Education, Perth, WA.

Dubé, V., Ducharme, F., 2015. Nursing reflective practice: an empirical literature review. J. Nurs. Educ. Pract. 5 (7), 91–99.

Egan, R., Testa, D., 2010. Models of supervision. In: Stagnitti, K., Schoo, A., Welch, D. (Eds.), Clinical and Fieldwork Placement in the Health Professions. Oxford University Press, Melbourne, pp. 145–158.

Emden, C., Hutt, D., Bruce, M., 2003. Portfolio learning/ assessment in nursing and midwifery: an innovation in progress. Contemp. Nurse 16 (1–2), 124–132.

Fricke, M., 2015. Continuing competence program for the College of Physiotherapists of Manitoba. www .manitobaphysio.com/wp-content/uploads/Web-Continuin g-Competence-Program-Info-2015.pdf. (Accessed 3 June 2019).

Gaberson, K., Oermann, M.H. (Eds.), 2007. Clinical Teaching Strategies in Nursing. Springer, New York.

Gadbury-Amyot, C.C., Overman, P.R., 2018. Implementation of portfolios as a programmatic global assessment measure in dental education. J. Dent. Educ. 82 (6), 557–564.

Gadbury-Amyot, C.C., McCracken, D., Woldt, J.L., et al., 2014. Validity and reliability of portfolio assessment of student competence in two dental school populations: a four-year study. J. Dent. Educ. 78 (5), 657–667.

Gent, P., 2016. Continuing professional development for paramedics: a systematic literature review. Australas. J. Paramed. 13 (4).

Gibbs, G., Farmer, B., Eastcott, D., 1988. Learning by doing: a guide to teaching and learning methods. Further Education Unit, Oxford Polytechnic, Oxford, UK.

Green, J., Wyllie, A., Jackson, D., 2014. Electronic portfolios in nursing education: a review of the literature. Nurse Educ. Pract. 14 (1), 4–8.

Haldane, T., 2014. 'Portfolios' as a method of assessment in medical education. Gastroenterol. Hepatol. Bed Bench 7 (2), 89–93.

Hallam, G., Creagh, T., 2010. ePortfolio use by university students in Australia: a review of the Australian ePortfolio Project. High. Educ. Res. Dev. 29 (2), 179–193. https:// doi.org/10.1080/07294360903510582.

Hallam, G., Harper, W., McAllister, L., et al., 2010. Australian ePortfolio Project. ePortfolio use by university students in Australia: informing excellence in policy and practice. Supplementary report. Queensland University of Technology Department of eLearning Services, October. www.eportfoliopractice.qut.edu.au/survey/index.jsp. (Accessed 3 June 2019).

Health and Care Professions Council, 2014. Paramedics. https://www.hcpc-uk.org/aboutregistration/professions/ index.asp?id=10. (Accessed 7 April 2014).

Hoffman, T., Bennett, B., Del Mar, C., 2013. Evidence-Based Practice Across the Health Professions, second ed. Elsevier Australia, Sydney.

Hull, C., Redfern, L., Shuttleworth, A., 2005. Profiles and Portfolios: A Guide for Health and Social Care. Palgrave Macmillan, London.

Irby, B.J., 2012. Editor's overview: mentoring, tutoring, and coaching. Mentor. Tutoring 20 (3), 297–301.

Jasper, M., Fulton, J., 2005. Marking criteria for assessing practice-based portfolios at masters level. Nurse Educ. Today 25, 377–389.

Jasper, M., Rosser, M., Mooney, G.P., 2013. Professional Development, Reflection and Decision-Making in Nursing and Healthcare, second ed. John Wiley & Sons, Chichester.

Jessop, T., 2017. Inspiring transformation through TESTA's program approach. In: Carless, D., Bridges, S.M., Chan, C., et al. (Eds.), Scaling Up Assessment for Learning in Higher Education. Springer, Singapore, pp. 49–64.

Johnston, T., Acker, J., 2015. Embracing FOAMed for paramedic education. Response: J. Paramedics A'asia 42, 9–10.

Jones, L., Allen, B., Dunn, P., et al., 2017. Demystifying the rubric: a five-step pedagogy to improve student understanding and utilization of marking criteria. High. Educ. Res. Dev. 36 (1), 129–142.

Joyes, G., Gray, L., Hartnell-Young, E., 2010. Effective practice with e-portfolios: how can the UK experience inform implementation? Australas. J. Educ. Technol. 26 (1), 15–27.

Knowles, M.S., Holton, E.F., Swanson, R.A., 2015. The Adult Learner: The Definitive Classic in Adult Education and

Human Resource Development, eighth ed. Routledge, Abingdon-on-Thames.

Kolb, D., 1984. Experiential Learning: Experience as the Source of Learning and Development. Prentice-Hall, Englewood Cliffs, NJ.

Laux, M., Stoten, S., 2016. A statewide RN-BSN consortium use of the electronic portfolio to demonstrate student competency. Nurse Educ. 41 (6), 275–277.

Martin, J., 2006. The challenge of introducing continuous professional development for paramedics. J. Emerg. Prim. Health Care 4 (2).

MCEECDYA, 2010. The Australian blueprint for career development, prepared by Miles Morgan Australia, Commonwealth of Australia, Canberra. Available at: https://www.education.gov.au/australian-blueprint-career-development. (Accessed 28 May 2019).

Mills, J., 2009. Professional portfolios and Australian registered nurses requirements for licensure: developing an essential tool. Nurs. Health Sci. 11, 206–210.

Monash University, 2010. Sample critical incident report. www.monash.edu.au/lls/llonline/writing/medicine/reflective/5.xml. (Accessed 3 June 2019).

New Zealand Government, 2019. Health Practitioners Competence Assurance Act 2003. http://www.legislation.govt.nz/act/public/2003/0048/latest/DLM203312.html. (Accessed 10 April 2019).

Nickson, C.P., Cadogan, M.D., 2014. Free Open Access Medical education (FOAM) for the emergency physician. Emerg. Med. Australas. 26, 76–83.

Norman, K., 2008. Providing evidence of achievement. In: Norman, K. (Ed.), Portfolios in the Nursing Profession. Quay Books, London.

Nursing and Midwifery Board of Australia, 2014. Nurse practitioner standards for practice. Revised 2018. www.nursingmidwiferyboard.gov.au/Codes-Guidelines-Statements/Professional-standards/nurse-practitioner-standards-of-practice.aspx. (Accessed 10 April 2019).

Nursing and Midwifery Board of Australia (NMBA), 2016a. Australia: Registered nurse standards for practice. www.nursingmidwiferyboard.gov.au/News/2016-02-01-revised-standards.aspx. (Accessed 3 June 2019).

Nursing and Midwifery Board of Australia, 2016b. Enrolled nurse standards for practice. https://www.nursingmidwiferyboard.gov.au/Codes-Guidelines-Statements/Professional-standards/enrolled-nurse-standards-for-practice.aspx. (Accessed 3 June 2019).

Nursing and Midwifery Board of Australia (NMBA), 2016c. Registration standard: continuing professional development. https://www.nursingmidwiferyboard.gov.au/Registration-Standards/Continuing-professional-development.aspx. (Accessed 28 May 2019).

Nursing Council of New Zealand, 2017. Competencies for the nurse practitioner scope of practice. http://www.nursingcouncil.org.nz/Nurses/Scopes-of-practice/Nurse-practitioner. (Accessed 10 April 2019).

Occupational Therapy Board of Australia, 2012. Continuing professional development (CPD) registration standard. https://www.occupationaltherapyboard.gov.au/Registration-Standards/Continuing-professional-development.aspx. (Accessed 3 June 2019).

O'Connell, J., Gardner, G., Coyer, F., 2014. Beyond competencies: using a capability framework in developing practice standards for advanced practice nursing. J. Adv. Nurs. 70 (12), 2728–2735.

Office of the Australian Information Commissioner, 2019. Privacy, https://www.oaic.gov.au/privacy. (Accessed 10 April 2019).

O'Meara, P.F., Furness, S., Gleeson, R., 2017. Educating paramedics in the future: a holistic approach. J. Health Hum. Serv. Adm. 40 (2), 219–251.

Paramedicine Board of Australia, 2018a. Regulating Australia's paramedics. https://www.paramedicineboard.gov.au/. (Accessed 24 May 2019).

Paramedicine Board of Australia, 2018b. Continuing professional development. https://www.paramedicineboard.gov.au/Professional-standards/Registration-standards/CPD.aspx#_blank. (Accessed 24 May 2019).

Paramedics Australasia, 2016. New Zealand moves ahead with paramedic registration. https://www.paramedics.org/new-zealand-moves-ahead-with-paramedic-registration-2/. (Accessed 24 May 2019).

Paramedicine Board of Australia, 2019. Professional capabilities for registered paramedics. https://www.paramedicineboard.gov.au/Professional-standards/Professional-capabilities-for-registered-paramedics.aspx. (Accessed 23 September 2019).

Pearce, R., 2003. Profiles and Portfolios of Evidence. Nelson Thornes, Cheltenham, UK.

Pharmacy Board of Australia, 2014. National competency standards framework for pharmacists in Australia. www.pharmacyboard.gov.au/Registration-Standards.aspx. (Accessed 1 February 2016).

Pharmacy Board of Australia, 2015a. Guidelines on continuing professional development. www.pharmacyboard.gov.au/Codes-Guidelines.aspx. (Accessed 3 June 2019).

Pharmacy Board of Australia, 2015b. Recency of practice registration standard. www.pharmacyboard.gov.au/Registration-Standards.aspx. (Accessed 3 June 2019).

Prehospital and Retrieval Medicine, 2015. Ketamine: how to use it fearlessly for all its indications. http://prehospitalmed.com/2015/12/04/ketamine-how-to-use-it-fearlessly-for-all-its-indications-by-strayer. (Accessed 3 June 2019).

Privacy Commissioner New Zealand, 2019. https://www.privacy.org.nz/. (Accessed 1 July 2019).

Reeves, S., Perrier, L., Goldman, J., et al., 2013. Interprofessional education: effects on professional practice and healthcare outcomes. Cochrane Database Syst. Rev. (3), CD002213, https://doi.org/10.1002/14651858.CD002213.pub3.

Scholes, J., Webb, J., Gray, M., et al., 2004. Making portfolios work in practice. J. Adv. Nurs. 46 (6), 595–603.

Schuster, P.M., 2008. Concept Mapping: A Critical Thinking Approach to Care Planning. FA Davis, Philadelphia, PA.

Sezer, D., Anderson, L., O'Reilly, M., et al., 2015. Assessing interprofessional competence using a prospective reflective portfolio. J. Interprof. Care 29 (3), 179–187.

Taylor, B., 2006. Reflective practice: a guide for nurses and midwives. Open University Press, London.

Taylor, M., Hill, S., 2014. Consumer expectations and healthcare in Australia. Deeble Institute for Health Policy Research, Australian Healthcare and Hospitals Association, Canberra.

Tolari, T., Acker, J., 2013. The national registration of paramedics: the ride to the future: is it better late than never? Response: J. Paramed. Australas. 20, 13–15.

Wiliam, D., 2013. Assessment: the bridge between teaching and learning. Voices from the Middle 21 (2), 15–20. www.ncte.org/library/NCTEFiles/Resources/Journals/VM/0212-dec2013/VM0212Assessment.pdf. (Accessed 3 June 2019).

Glossary

Australian Health Practitioner Regulation Agency (AHPRA) The organisation responsible for the implementation of the National Registration and Accreditation Scheme across Australia through the various National Health Practitioner Boards.

The 15 Boards include:

- Aboriginal and Torres Strait Islander Health Practice Board of Australia
- Chinese Medicine Board of Australia
- Chiropractic Board of Australia
- Dental Board of Australia
- Medical Board of Australia
- Medical Radiation Practice Board of Australia
- Nursing and Midwifery Board of Australia
- Occupational Therapy Board of Australia
- Optometry Board of Australia
- Osteopathy Board of Australia
- Paramedicine Board of Australia
- Pharmacy Board of Australia
- Physiotherapy Board of Australia
- Podiatry Board of Australia
- Psychology Board of Australia.

AHPRA's operations are governed by the Health Practitioner Regulation National Law.

AHPRA supports the 15 National Boards that are responsible for regulating the health professions under the National Registration and Accreditation Scheme.

Australian Nursing and Midwifery Accreditation Council (ANMAC) The independent accrediting authority for the Nursing and Midwifery Board of Australia under the National Registration and Accreditation Scheme. ANMAC develops standards for accreditation and accredits nursing and midwifery courses and providers.

Autonomy Having a sense of one's own identity and an ability to act independently and to exert control over one's environment, including a sense of task mastery, internal locus of control and self-efficacy.

Client/patient A person or persons who engage(s) or is/are served by the professional advice or services of another. May refer to an individual, family or community. Use of 'client' acknowledges that a significant proportion of nursing services are delivered to people who are well and proactively engaging in healthcare. Use of 'patient' acknowledges that nursing provides some of its services to people who are sick and, in the true Latin meaning, are 'suffering'. However, 'client' and 'patient' are used synonymously to acknowledge that the same services may be used for both clients and patients.

e-Portfolios The use of online or electronic technologies to achieve the same aims as other forms of portfolio.

Evidence Objective and subjective information that forms the basis of a portfolio. Portfolio evidence may take different forms, including objects, statements, documents, recordings and other products that demonstrate and support the achievements and claims.

Lifelong learning A full and successful life, including effective work performance, requires continued openness to, and participation in, education and learning. This learning may take place through a range of sources, from university and vocational formal qualifications to other types of programs, courses and events, as well as on-the-job training and personal and informal learning.

Performance assessment Measurement against professional, educational and/or organisational criteria of how an individual uses their knowledge and skills to produce or complete the required level of performance.

Portfolios Compilation of a portfolio requires purposeful selection and structuring of different types of evidence to meet specific goals. These may include individual professional goals, competencies, career achievements and continuing professional development activities and experiences. A portfolio may be developed for education, certification, employment or promotion purposes. Depending on the specific purpose, a portfolio may highlight only best-practice examples of competency and performance-based achievements, as well as a summative evaluation of strengths and weaknesses, or it may also include 'works in progress' that show development and improvement over time.

Reflective practice A way of learning that involves using personal experience as a basis from which to identify and understand the knowledge that is developed from and used in practice.

Reliability The extent to which a tool will function consistently in the same way with repeated use.

Scopes of practice The complete range of roles, functions, responsibilities, activities and decision-making abilities that a health practitioner is qualified, competent and authorised by legislation, regulation and employers to perform.

Validity The extent to which a measurement tool measures what it purports to measure.

Web-folio A portfolio displayed as a website, with a combination of headings, text explanations and embedded digital artefacts to provide evidence to support the claims being made.

Index

Page numbers followed by 'f' indicate figures, 't' indicate tables, and 'b' indicate boxes.

A

academic records, 80
accountability, 32, 37
accreditation, 73–74
achievement portfolio, 74
  assessment of, 74
  product/achievement portfolio, 74
action plan, 40
adult learning, concept of, 10
AHPRA *see* Australian Health Practitioner Regulation Agency
analysis, in portfolio development, 28t
anxiety disorders, 36b–37b
appendices, in framework, 64–65, 65b
applicant feedback, 81–84
application, in portfolio development, 28t
argument, 3, 37, 63
artefacts, as primary evidence, 53
assessment
  assessor, 73
  basic assumptions about, 73
  criterion-referenced, 80
  to direct and stimulate learning, 77–78
  of document, 48
  for employment, 78–79, 79b
  evidence, 48
  feedback and, 73
  formative, 81
  grades awarded in, 80
  moderation, 81
  norm-referenced, 80
  of outcomes, 77t, 77b
  outset of, 79
  of performance, 53
  portfolio approaches and impact on, 73–74
  portfolio evaluation and, 74–79
  practice standards, 69t–71t
  quality, 73
  rubric, 80–81, 81t–82t
  student/applicant feedback, 81–84
  summative, 81–84
  supporting student learning through, 84–85
  validity and reliability of, 85
assessor, 73
audience, of portfolio, 17–18, 24
audit results, 52–53
Australia, paramedics in, 106
Australian Coalition of National Nursing Organisations, members of, 9t
Australian College of Pharmacy (ACP), 112
Australian Health Practitioner Regulation Agency (AHPRA), 6

B

best practice, shared models of, 54–55
blog entry, 39–40, 40f
brainstorming, 42–43

C

calculations, associated, 80
capability, 2
career development, 12
career planning
  portfolios for, 12
  steps in, 12
case studies, 48, 54, 64–65
clinical/practice situation, learning from, 38–39
clusters, 42–43
collective competence, 54–55
communicating competence, 6
  for enrolled nurse practice, 100, 100t–101t
  health workforce in, 2
  for midwifery practice, 91–93, 91t
  for midwives, registered nurses and enrolled nurses, 89–90
  in occupational therapy, 102–103, 103t
  in paramedicine, 106–109
  in pharmacy, 110–113
  professional development in, 6–7
  professional practice in, regulation of, 6
  for registered nurse practice, 94–99
communication, practice standards, 69t–71t
communicator, 11
competence
  collective, 54–55
  communicating, 6
  inter-professional and team, 54
competency
  collective, 54–55
  domain, 64–65
  levels of, 50
  standards, 64–65

compiling, of portfolios, 16–17, 61–71
  collecting information or evidence, 65–67, 66t
  confidentiality in, 19
  framework for, 62–65, 66t
    appendices, 64–65, 65b
    design, 62
    personal details, 62–63
    statement of learning, 63–64
  and generating new evidence, 67–71, 69t–71t
  identifying omissions in, 67–71, 69t–71t
  over time, 78
  privacy in, 19
  steps in, 61–62
  suggested, 62–65
  template for, 66t
comprehension, in portfolio development, 28t
concept maps
  for reflection, 42–44, 42f–43f, 44b
  software, 23
confidentiality
  of evidence, 55
  portfolio and, 19
connections, 3
consent, 53
contextually aware, 11
continuing professional development (CPD), 6–7
  activities for, evaluation of, 92–93, 92t–93t
  activity groups, 111t
  for pharmacists, 111–112
  planning for, 102–103
    and evaluation, health practitioners' approaches to, 88–113
    examples of, 102, 104t–105t
    in pharmacy, 110–111
  requirements for, 89
  structured approach to, 106–109
course-related portfolio, 63
CPD see continuing professional development
criterion-referenced assessment, 80
critical incident analysis, 40

D

deeper levels of meaning, 38
delivery of care, practice standards, 69t–71t
depression, 36b–37b
design, framework for, 62
development, portfolio, 27–29, 28t
discipline-based knowledge, 32–34
disclosure, 19, 53
display function, in e-portfolio, 24–25
documents
  assessment, 48
  institutional, 65
  PDF and Word, 23

as primary evidence, 53
regulatory, 67

E

education
  collective competence and, 54–55
  portfolio in, 2
e-gimmickry, 27
e-learning, 21
electronic portfolios, 10
employing organisations, 8
employment, 11
  assessment for, 78–79, 79b
engaging others
  how to, 45–46
  reasons for, 45
  in reflection, 44–46, 45f
  rules of, 46
enrolled nurse practice, communicating competence, 100, 100t–101t
enrolled nurses, communicating competence for, 89–90
e-portfolio, 12, 16–17, 27b
  benefits of, 27b
  challenges in, 27b
  components of, 21–22, 21f
  display function in, 24–25
  e-learning and, 21
  e-tools in, 22–23, 22b
  issues with, 25–27
  limitations of, 25–27
  organisation of, 20–27
  platform, 23
  potential risks of, 27b
  presentation of, 20–27
  in promotion application, 27, 28t
  reflection and, 20–21
  tagging in, 23–24
  terms, 21
  web-folio, 21, 24
ethics, 34
e-tools, 22–23, 22b
evaluation
  in portfolio development, 28t
  practice standards, 69t–71t
evidence, 47–60
  appendices, 64–65, 65b
  collecting, 65–67
  compiling portfolios and, 67–71, 69t–71t
  complexity of, 2
  confidentiality of, 55
  healthcare decisions based on, 52
  meaningful, 52
    relevancy of, 55
    suitability of, 55

evidence *(Continued)*
  new, generating, 67–71
  omissions in, 67–71
  for portfolio, 55–57, 56*t*, 56*b*
  pre-existing, 67
  primary, 53, 65
  privacy and, 53, 55
  in professional portfolio, 3
  purpose of, 48–50, 51*b*
    assessment, 48
    starting point for, 48
  quality of, 51–55, 55*b*
  range of, 57–60, 58*b*–59*b*, 59*f*–60*f*, 68
  research, 49–50
  secondary, 53, 65
  selecting, 57, 57*b*
  selection and use of, 50
  sources, range of, 54–55
  structure and, 75*t*–76*t*
  summary table of, 64, 64*t*
  tangible, 51–53
  types of, 49*f*
    healthcare decisions based on, 49–50
evidence-based healthcare, 52
evidence-based practice, 49–50
experiential learning approach, 34–35, 35*f*,
      35*b*–37*b*
experiential placements, note-taking and, 54
explanation, 48–49

F

feedback
  assessment and, 73
  as exchange, 46
  quality, 46
  student/applicant, 81–84
'feedback sheets', 80–81
formal knowledge, 32–34
formal learning, 35
formative assessment, 81
framework, for compiling portfolios, 3, 62–65, 66*t*
  appendices, 64–65, 65*b*
  competency domain, 65
  evidence summary table, 64, 64*t*
  personal details, 62–63
  standard or competency domain, 3
  statement of justification, 63
  statement of learning, 63–64
  summary statement of arguments or claims, 63
  template, 66*t*
Free Open Access Medical education (FOAMed),
      109
'frontload' learning, 77–78

G

generic skills *see* process skills
Gibbs reflective cycle, 39–40, 40*f*, 41*b*
goal-setting, 12
grades, awarding, 80
'grading schemes', 80–81
group work, 45

H

*Health Practitioner Regulation National Law Act
      2009*, 6
health practitioners
  career planning for, 11–12
  lifelong learning skills in, 10–11
  portfolio in, 1
  privacy, confidentiality and disclosure, 19
  regulation, websites for, 7*b*–8*b*
  regulatory authorities of, 2
  statutory regulation of, 6
Health Practitioners Competence Assurance Act, 52
healthcare
  changes in, 11–12
  evidence-based, 49–50, 52
honesty, 38

I

idea-generation, 42–43
identification, in portfolio development, 28*t*
individual accountability, 32
informal learning, 35
information, collecting, 65–67, 66*t*
information clustering, 42–43
information literate, 10
institutional documents, 65
intended audience, of portfolio, 17–18
intended portfolio outcomes, 77*t*, 77*b*
intent, 53
inter-professional competence, 54

J

job description, 17
job promotion, portfolio for, 27, 28*t*
journal, reflective, 39–40, 40*f*
justification, statement of, 63

K

knowledge, 11
  discipline-based, 32–34
Kolb, David, 34

L

learning
  activities, for paramedics, 107–109, 108t–109t
    needs, self-identification of, 110
    outcomes, 109
  assessing to direct and stimulate, 77–78
  from clinical/practice situation, 38–39
  by doing, 31–32
  e-learning, 21
  experiential approach, 34–35, 35f, 35b–37b
  formal, 35
  'frontload', 77–78
  informal, 35
  lifelong, 10–11
  plan, development of, 106–107
  reflective, 30–31, 34–35
  supporting, through assessment, 84–85
learning portfolio see process-oriented portfolio
letters, reference, 53
Lewin, Kurt, 35, 35f
lifelong learning, reflection and, 10–11, 11b
log, of activities, 103

M

Medicines Safety Update, 112
merit-based grades, 85
midwives, communicating competence for, 89–90
models
  best practice, 54–55
  portfolio, 15–29, 29b
moderation processes, 81
multiple documents, in portfolios, 5

N

National Board, 6
'National Law', 6
netiquette, 26
new evidence, generating, 67–71
New Zealand, paramedics in, 106
NMBA see Nursing and Midwifery Board of Australia
NMBA Nursing and Midwifery Continuing Professional
    Development Registration Standard, 43–44
non-graded pass/fail see criterion-referenced assessment
norm-referenced assessment, 80
notes
  in clinical or experiential placements, 54
  for compiling portfolios, 67
NPS Medicineswise, 112
nurse practitioner status, application for, portfolio in,
    27, 29t
nursing, process of, 42, 42f

Nursing and Midwifery Board of Australia (NMBA), 89
  enrolled nurse standards for practice, 100

O

objectivity, 38
occupational therapists, registration renewal for, 102
occupational therapy, communicating competence in,
    102–103, 103t
omissions, evidence, 67–71
organisation, of portfolio, 19–27, 75t–76t
organisational sense, portfolio in, 3
organisations, professional, 2, 8
outcomes, learning, 109

P

paper-based portfolios, 16–17
paramedicine
  in Australia and New Zealand, 106
  communicating competence for, 106–109
Paramedics Australasia, 106
peer appraisal, 45
performance assessment, 53
personal details, 62–63
personal development, 69t–71t
personal reflective statements, 5
personal understandings, 32–34
Pharmaceutical Society of Australia (PSA), 112
pharmacists
  continuing professional development available for, 111–112
  continuing professional development for, 110
  scope of practice for, 110–111
pharmacy, communicating competence for practice in,
    110–113
Pharmacy Board of Australia (PharmBA), 110
  continuing professional development plan template from,
    112
  frequently asked questions, 111–112
  standards and guidelines, 110
Pharmacy Guild of Australia (PGA), 112
photographs, 52–53
placements, clinical or experiential, 54
platform, e-portfolio, 23
political sense, portfolio in, 3
portable document format (PDF), 16–17
'portfolio defence', 85
portfolios, 1–14, 3b–4b, 10b, 13b–14b, 77–78, 86b
  appearance of, 15–18, 18b
  approaches and impact on assessment, 73–74, 74b
  assessment, 77t, 77b
    and evaluation, 74–79
    outcomes, 78–79, 79b
    of product/achievement, 74

portfolios *(Continued)*
    in broader curriculum, 78
    building, 18*b*
    and career planning, 11–12, 13*b*
    challenges of, 27*b*
    compiling of, 61–71 *see also* compiling, of portfolios
        evidence and, 67–71, 69*t*–71*t*
        steps in, 61–62
        template for, 66*t*
    components of, 5*f*
    course-related, 63
    definition of, 3–4
    development and use of, steps and responsibilities in
        27–29, 28*t*
    e-portfolio, 5, 10, 16–17, 27*b*
        benefits of, 27*b*
        challenges in, 27*b*
        components of, 21–22, 21*f*
        display function in, 24–25
        e-learning and, 21
        e-tools in, 22–23, 22*b*
        issues with, 25–27
        limitations of, 25–27
        organisation of, 20–27
        platform, 23
        potential risks of, 27*b*
        presentation of, 20–27
        reflection and, 20–21
        tagging, 23–24
        terms, 21
        web-folio, 21, 24
    electronic, 10
    evidences for, 55–57, 56*t*, 56*b*
    forms of, 4–8, 4*b*–5*b*
    importance of, 1–2
    as learning workspace, 16
    models of, 15–29, 29*b*
    for nurse practitioner status, 27, 29*t*
    organisation, 19–27, 75*t*–76*t*
    potential risks of, 27*b*
    presentation of, 19–27
    process-oriented, 73–74, 75*t*–76*t*
    producing, 79
    product-oriented, 73–74, 75*t*–76*t*
    professional, 75*t*–76*t*
    purpose of, 18, 75*t*–76*t*
    quality of, 48
    reflection and, 30–31, 37
    regulation requirements for, 8, 8*b*
    selecting evidence for, 57
    as showcase, 16
    specific purpose of, 48–50, 51*b*
    standards-based, 63
    structure of, 19–20, 20*b*, 29*b*, 75*t*–76*t*
    styles of, 15–29

    table of contents of, 61
    value of, 37
    see also assessment; evidence
practice standards, 69*t*–71*t*
Prehospital and Retrieval Medicine (PHARM), 109
preparation, necessary for reflection, 38
presentation, of portfolios, 19–27
primary evidence, 53, 65
privacy
    evidence and, 53, 55
    portfolio and, 19
process-oriented portfolio, 73–74, 75*t*–76*t*
process skills, 34
product-oriented portfolio, 73–74, 75*t*–76*t*
profession, practice standards, 69*t*–71*t*
professional development, continuing, 6–7
professional development plan, 92
    evaluation of, 94–99, 95*t*–98*t*, 112
    key questions to be addressed in, 112
    paramedic, planning and recording of, 106
professional organisations, 8
professional portfolios, 1–14, 3*b*
    approaches, 75*t*–76*t*
    see also portfolios
professional practice
    reflection meaning and uses for, 30–31
    regulation of, 6–7
purpose
    of assessment, 72–73
    of evidence, 48–50, 51*b*
    of portfolio, 18, 75*t*–76*t*
    of reflection, 32
    statement, 42–43

Q

quality
    of assessment, 73
    of evidence, 51–55, 55*b*
    of feedback, 46
    of portfolio, 51–55
    of secondary evidence, 53

R

recognition, in portfolio development, 28*t*
records, academic, 80
reference letter, 53
reflection, 17–18, 109
    analytical aspects of, 31
    broad approaches in, 38
    concept maps for, 42–44, 42*f*–43*f*, 44*b*
    conditions necessary for, 38
    critical incident analysis as, 40
    engaging others in, 44–46, 45*f*

focused approaches in, 38
on learning from clinical/practice situation, 38
levels of, 40
lifelong learning and, 10–11, 11*b*
meaning and uses of, 30–31
portfolios and, 30–31, 37
process of, 31
purpose of, 32
reflective learning and, 34–35
terminology of, 30–31
tools for, 37–46, 41*b*
writing, 39–40
reflective cycle, Gibbs, 39–40, 40*f*, 41*b*
reflective journal, 39–40, 40*f*
reflective learning, 34–35
reflective practice, 31–32
reflective practitioner, 32–34, 32*b*–33*b*
reflective processes, 11
reflective statements, personal, 5
reflective thinking, fundamental aspect of, 32
reflexivity, 109
registered nurse practice, communicating competence for, 94–99
registered nurses, communicating competence for, 89–90
registration standards, 6
regulation, statutory, of health practitioners, 6
regulatory documents, 67
relevant evidence, 55
reliability, of assessment, 85
research evidence, 49–50
rubric, assessment, 80–81, 81*t*–82*t*
rules of engagement, 46

S

schema, assessment, 79
scopes of practice, for pharmacists, 110–111
'scoring guides', 80–81
secondary evidence, 53, 65
self-awareness, 12
showcase, quality portfolio as, 37
social networking, 26
Society of Hospital Pharmacists of Australia (SHPA), 111
software programs, e-portfolio, 21, 24
sources, range of, 54–55
standards
  competency, 64–65
  domain, 64–65
  in portfolios, 3
  practice, 55, 69*t*–71*t*
  of practice, 2

statement
  of justification, 63
  purpose, 42–43
  summary, of arguments or claims, 63
storage space, quality portfolio as, 37
'strengths, weaknesses, opportunities and threats (SWOT)' analysis, 39
structure
  evidence and, 75*t*–76*t*
  portfolio, 19–20, 20*b*, 29*b*, 75*t*–76*t*
student feedback, 81–84
suggested framework, for portfolio, 62–65
suitable evidence, 55
summary statement, of arguments or claims, 63
summary table, of evidence, 64, 64*t*
summative assessment, 81–84
SWOT analysis, 39
synthesis, in portfolio development, 28*t*

T

table of contents, in compiling portfolio, 61
tagging, in e-portfolio, 23–24
tangible evidence, 51–53
team competence, 54
technology, 10
template, for framework, 66*t*
tools
  e-tools, 22–23, 22*b*
  for reflection, 37–46, 41*b*

U

understanding, necessary for reflection, 38

V

validity, of assessment, 85
voluminous portfolio, 20

W

web-folio, 21, 24
wiki, 22
Word files, PDF compared with, 26
workplace context, 50
workspace, quality portfolio as, 37
World Alliance for Patient Safety, 2
writing, reflective, 39–40
written consent, 55